Simplified
TAI CHI CHUAN

Simplified
TAI CHI CHUAN

24 Postures

with Applications
AND

Standard
48 Postures

太極拳與應用

LIANG, SHOU-YU AND WU, WEN-CHING

YMAA Publication Center, Inc.
Wolfeboro, NH USA

YMAA Publication Center, Inc.
PO Box 480
Wolfeboro, NH 03894
800 669 8892 • www.ymaa.com • info@ymaa.com

Paperback
ISBN: 9781594392788

Ebook
ISBN: 9781594392795

Enhanced Ebook
ISBN: 9781594392917

Second edition, revised. Copyright ©1993, 1996, 2014 by Liang, Shou-Yu and Wu, Wen-Ching

Cover design by Axie Breen

Copyedit by Dolores Sparrow and T. G. LaFredo

Proofreading by Sara Scanlon • Indexing by Susan Bullowa

Photos by YMAA unless noted otherwise.

Figures on pages 39, 40, 43, 45, and 47 modified by Axie Breen from original images copyright ©1994 by TechPool Studios Corp. USA, 1463 Warrensville Center Road, Cleveland, OH 44121.

10 9 8 7 6 5 4 3 2

Publisher's Cataloging in Publication

Liang, Shou-Yu, 1943-

    Simplified tai chi chuan : 24 postures with applications and standard 48 postures / Liang, Shou-Yu and Wen-Ching Wu. -- Second edition, revised. -- Wolfeboro, NH : YMAA Publication Center, c2014.

    p. ; cm.

    ISBN: 978-1-59439-278-8 (pbk.) ; 978-1-59439-279-5 (ebk.) ; 978-1-59439-291-7 (enh. ebk.)

    Revises the 1996 second edition, issued as: Tai chi chuan: 24 and 48 postures with martial applications.

    Includes bibliographical references and index.

    Summary: This book is designed for self-study and can help you learn both the Simplified Tai Chi 24 Posture form and the Simplified Tai Chi Chuan 48 Posture form quickly and accurately. With a new and easy-to-follow layout, every movement is presented in 2-4 large photos with 'to the point' instructions.--Publisher.

    1. Tai chi. 2. Qi (Chinese philosophy) 3. Mind and body. 4. Martial arts. I. Wu, Wen-Ching, 1964- II. Title. III. Title: Tai chi chuan: 24 and 48 postures with martial applications.

GV504 .L487 2014   2014930327
613.7/148--dc23   1405

The practice, treatments, and methods described in this book should not be used as an alternative to professional medical diagnosis or treatment. The authors and publisher of this book are NOT RESPONSIBLE in any manner whatsoever for any injury or negative effects that may occur through following the instructions and advice contained herein.

It is recommended that before beginning any treatment or exercise program, you consult your medical professional to determine whether you should undertake this course of practice.

Warning: While self-defense is legal, fighting is illegal. If you don't know the difference, you'll go to jail because you aren't defending yourself. You are fighting—or worse. Readers are encouraged to be aware of all appropriate local and national laws relating to self-defense, reasonable force, and the use of weaponry, and to act in accordance with all applicable laws at all times. Understand that while legal definitions and interpretations are generally uniform, there are small—but very important—differences from state to state and even city to city. To stay out of jail, you need to know these differences. Neither the authors nor the publisher assumes any responsibility for the use or misuse of information contained in this book.

Nothing in this document constitutes a legal opinion, nor should any of its contents be treated as such. While the authors believe everything herein is accurate, any questions regarding specific self-defense situations, legal liability, and/or interpretation of federal, state, or local laws should always be addressed by an attorney at law.

When it comes to martial arts, self-defense, and related topics, no text, no matter how well written, can substitute for professional, hands-on instruction. These materials should be used for academic study only.

Printed in Canada.

Editorial Notes

Romanization of Chinese Words

The interior of this book primarily uses the Pinyin romanization system of Chinese to English. In some instances, a more popular word may be used as an aid for reader convenience, such as "tai chi" in place of the Pinyin spelling, *taiji*. Pinyin is standard in the People's Republic of China and in several world organizations, including the United Nations. Pinyin, which was introduced in China in the 1950s, replaces the older Wade-Giles and Yale systems.

Some common conversions are found in the following:

Pinyin	Also spelled as	Pronunciation
qi	chi	chē
qigong	chi kung	chē gōng
qin na	chin na	chǐn nǎ
jin	jing	jǐn
gongfu	kung fu	gōng foo
taijiquan	tai chi chuan	tī jē chǔén

For more information, please refer to *The People's Republic of China: Administrative Atlas, The Reform of the Chinese Written Language,* or a contemporary manual of style.

Formats and Treatment of Chinese Words

The first instances of foreign words in the text proper are set in italics. Transliterations are provided frequently: for example, Eight Pieces of Brocade (Ba Duan Jin, 八段錦).

Chinese persons' names are mostly presented in their more popular English spelling. Capitalization is according to the *Chicago Manual of Style* 16th edition. The author or publisher may use a specific spelling or capitalization in respect to the living or deceased person. For example: Cheng, Man-ch'ing can be written as Zheng Manqing.

Photographs

Many photographs include motion arrows to help show the starting position of the body motion. Front view, rear view, or mirror image photographs are occasionally used as an additional aid for posture movements.

Table of Contents

Foreword by Grandmaster Wang, Ju-Rong

Taijiquan (tai chi chuan) is a "blooming flower" among today's "garden" of Chinese *wushu* styles. It has been under constant refinement and enrichment over the long history of Chinese martial arts development. It is like an "old branch blossoming with new flowers." Its "fragrance" flows far and wide, over the oceans and over the mountain peaks, to become an international health-strengthening exercise. People are becoming familiar with taijiquan and are falling in love with it.

Since Chen, Yang, Wǔ, Wu, and Sun—the five major taijiquan styles—became known to the world, many new sequences have been compiled. Among them are the 24 and the 48 Posture Taijiquan, which have received broad acclaim both in and outside of China. They have been meritorious in promoting and developing taijiquan since the 1950s. Both sequences have paved the way for millions of taijiquan enthusiasts to enter the "broad palace" of taijiquan by erasing its mysterious, complex, monotonous, and obscure appearance. All over Chinese cities and countrysides, people are practicing the 24 and 48 Posture Taijiquan. Public health, education, and physical education departments all include taijiquan as an important part of their curriculum. Many nations and areas all over the world, including Japan, the United States, Europe, and Southeast Asia, all have taijiquan activities. Many nations have established taijiquan organizations, and periodically return to China to learn and to share their experience.

Chinese wushu includes unique offensive and defensive martial applications. Taijiquan also has unique characteristics in its applications. This is the essence included in the intriguing taijiquan push hands training: it uses steadiness against motion, it uses yielding against force, it avoids frontal confrontation and attacks the insubstantial, and it borrows the opponent's power to emit power.

We have here Coach Liang, Shou-Yu, a multitalented Chinese martial arts expert and famous martial arts coach currently residing in Canada, and Coach Wu, Wen-Ching, an outstanding young martial artist and a national competition grand champion: both cooperating to promote taijiquan. They have not limited their contribution to teaching the different styles of taijiquan. They have now completed *Simplified Tai Chi Chuan: 24 and 48 Postures with Martial Applications*. This book presents to interested readers many practical martial arts applications along with the health-promoting exercise of taijiquan. The combination of martial applications and health-promoting exercises will complement each other, making the taijiquan training more complete. This is a wonderful addition that brings to light the glory of the Chinese wushu tradition. It is a great pleasure to write the foreword for this book. I would also like to express my congratulations to Coach Liang and Coach Wu for a meticulous and successful cooperative effort in finishing this book.

Wang, Ju-Rong
Professor, China Shanghai Athletic Institute
Chinese Wushu National Level Judge

Foreword by
Dr. Yang, Jwing-Ming

After thousands of years of development, many different styles of taijiquan have been created. Although taijiquan was originally created as a martial art, it has continuously demonstrated its value in bringing the practitioner physical and spiritual health. Today, there are countless numbers of people, all over the world, who practice taijiquan purely for health. Many Western doctors are even recommending taijiquan to their patients to help lower high blood pressure, reduce stress, and to ease the tension of the internal organs. I deeply believe that taijiquan is on its way to becoming more popular and accepted in the Western world.

Practicing traditional taijiquan is a long process, requiring a lot of time, patience, and money. This is made difficult with the reality of today's hectic lifestyles. In order to ease the practice and study of taijiquan, traditional taijiquan was revised into shorter versions, including a 24 Posture and 48 Posture Taijiquan. Each of these sequences requires less time to learn and practice than the traditional 108 Posture long sequence. To a taijiquan beginner with little or no knowledge about taijiquan, these short sequences are a good start before committing to further study. From these two short sequences, a beginner will be able to grasp the basic concept of taijiquan, understand its theories, and most important of all, begin to feel the added relaxation and the spirit of the art.

I have known Master Liang, Shou-Yu for nearly eight years. During this period, we have freely shared our knowledge with each other. In my opinion, Master Liang has reached a very high level of proficiency in Chinese martial arts and *qigong*. Truly, he is a precious treasure in the modern martial arts world. Although I have been involved in Chinese martial arts and qigong for more than thirty years, compared to Master Liang, I feel that I am just a beginner. Presently, I am learning Xingyiquan and Baguazhang from Master Liang. These are some of the styles I have always wanted to learn since I was a child. To help publicize these two arts, Master Liang and I have published a book entitled *Hsing Yi Chuan*. Currently, together with Mr. Wu, Wen-Ching, we are working on the book *Emei Baguazhang*. We hope that through our efforts we can bring the Chinese martial arts culture into the Western world in an accurate and dignified manner.

Mr. Wu has been my student for nearly ten years. He is also one of the few disciples I have accepted. Although he lived in Africa with his family since the age of eleven, he continues to carry the Chinese virtues in his heart. In the last ten years of practicing with Master Liang and me, Mr. Wu has reached a good level of understanding of Chinese martial arts. I hope that through writing this book with Master Liang and with continual training and research, he will be able to reach a deeper understanding of the Chinese arts, as well as the meaning of life.

Finally, I strongly recommend this book to any taijiquan beginner. The unique part of this book, besides the movements of the postures, is the addition of the martial arts applications of each posture. Very often I see that in practicing these shorter taijiquan sequences, the martial arts applications are not emphasized. I personally believe that without the martial arts understanding, the practice of taijiquan would lose the essence and the original meaning of the art. I am confident that this book will direct you to successful taijiquan training, and to a healthy, long life.

Dr. Yang, Jwing-Ming
Boston, 1993

Preface by Mr. Wu, Wen-Ching
(First Edition, 1993)

Like most other youngsters, I perceived taijiquan (tai chi chuan) as an old person's exercise when I was growing up. It was "mysterious" and "strange," yet also "magical." It was inconceivable to me that I would later practice taijiquan, and even harder to imagine that I would become a taijiquan instructor. It was not until the fall of 1983 that I was introduced to the true potential of taijiquan by my *shifu* (teacher/father), Dr. Yang, Jwing-Ming. Ever since, my fascination and love for this ancient art has become the focal point of my life. The inner discipline of my martial arts training has significantly influenced my perspective on life. It has become more than martial arts training; it has opened my eyes to the endless potential of the *Dao* (*Tao*).

Teaching is learning, and it has been a way to further my understanding and training. Teaching has helped me learn how to communicate and explain clearly. The many years that I observed and assisted my teacher in teaching his classes at YMAA Headquarters have taught me how to present and explain information. The goal for my next stage of learning was to be able to present information on paper and share with others the many benefits that I have received from my teachers. When my *shibo* (teacher/older uncle), Master Liang, Shou-Yu, and Dr. Yang gave me the opportunity to coauthor this book, I was left speechless. Writing this book has not only cleared up any questions I had concerning taijiquan, it has also taught me how to organize and present written material better.

It is our intent in writing this book that it be easy to read and understand. All hard-to-understand terms will be explained in simple and easy phrases. It can be used as a learning tool as well as a book with high entertainment value. It is our hope that this book will clarify the common misconceptions about taijiquan, including the "mystical" powers of *energy* (*qi*) in our bodies. To help readers gain a better understanding of the culture from which taijiquan evolved, we will also briefly explain some Chinese beliefs, famous books, well-known people, and common phrases leading to the formation of taijiquan. We hope with this information it will not only make this book more entertaining, but also bring to light why such an ancient art is valued in Chinese society and throughout the world today.

After over a year of research and writing, corresponding with Master Liang for corrections, comments, ideas, and editing, we finally are able to present this book to the readers. This book is divided into five chapters. In chapter one, we will introduce the background leading to the development of taijiquan. In chapter two, we will present the guidelines of taijiquan practices. In chapter three, we will present the exercises that will prepare you for learning the taijiquan sequence. In chapter four, we will present the entire 24 postures with key points and applications. Chapter five will consist of the 48 Posture Taijiquan, a more advanced taijiquan sequence. The appendix includes 24 and 48 posture names in English and Pinyin.

I would like to take this opportunity to give special thanks to Dr. Yang for his technical advice and for giving me the opportunity to carry on his lineage. Also, special thanks to Master Liang for the opportunity to coauthor this book and for sharing his vast knowledge with me. And, of course, a special thanks to Denise Breiter for her countless hours of discussion and editing, and for helping me to bridge Chinese culture and language with Western culture and English language. Last, but certainly not least, my sincere gratitude to all my friends and colleagues for helping me to make this book possible.

Wu, Wen-Ching

Preface by Master Liang, Shou-Yu (First Edition, 1993)

There are many styles of taijiquan throughout China. The five most popular ones are Chen, Yang, Wu, Wŭ, and Sun Taijiquan. Within each one of these Taijiquan styles are different training approaches. It is difficult to tell which is better or more correct.

In 1956, the experts in charge of the Chinese National Athletic Association compiled the 24 Posture Taijiquan sequence, and in 1976, they compiled the 48 Posture Taijiquan sequence. These two Taijiquan sequences were used as the prototypes for popularizing taijiquan. After many years, these two sequences have become very popular in China, as well as in many other countries. These two sequences are well liked because they are simple, easy to learn, pleasing to watch, and standardized. It only takes six minutes to do the 24 Posture Taijiquan sequence and twelve minutes to perform the 48 Posture Taijiquan sequence. These two Taijiquan sequences gained their popularity because they can be learned and performed in a short period of time.

For taijiquan enthusiasts, learning the 24 Posture Taijiquan is not difficult. It was edited by many taijiquan experts and the movements are very accurate. It takes about ten hours of instruction to complete the form. Practicing this sequence daily should be sufficient to maintain your health. With the 24 Posture Taijiquan as a foundation, you can further your study of taijiquan easily with the 48 Posture Taijiquan.

From my thirty-two years of experience in teaching taijiquan, I have found that people who are interested in advanced taijiquan training can learn any other style of taijiquan with little or no difficulty, with the 24 and 48 Posture Taijiquan as a foundation. Training taijiquan gives one better health, a way of self-defense, and a good pastime. Many taijiquan practitioners are not only experts in cultivating their body's energy, but are also martial arts experts. Of course, in today's society, most people are only interested in taijiquan for its health-promoting benefits. However, if you are aware of the actual applications of the movements, you will develop a deeper appreciation for this ancient healing/martial art. Every traditional taijiquan instructor will introduce the applications of the taijiquan postures, training methods, and pushing hands methods. Many people aren't aware that in the 24 Posture Taijiquan sequence there are also high levels of applications in each and every posture. In this book, besides introducing the 24 and 48 Posture Taijiquan movements, we will also introduce the martial applications of the 24 Posture Taijiquan. Due to compiling limitations, we will not include these applications for the 48 Posture Taijiquan in this book. However, once you are familiar with the 24 Posture Taijiquan application concepts, it will be easy for you to learn the 48 Posture Taijiquan applications.

There are so many people who have helped me to get where I am today. I don't have many opportunities to express my sincere gratitude, but I would like to give special thanks to the following individuals.

Master Wang, Ju-Rong, former chief judge of the Chinese National Taijiquan Competitions, for writing the foreword for this book. She is of the older generation in Chinese martial arts, and is the daughter of the most famous martial arts master in recent history, Master Wang, Zi-ping—the late head coach of the Shaolin Division in the Central Guoshu Institute, whom I have had the highest admiration and respect for ever since I was a child. Master Wang, Ju-Rong has given me much encouragement and support for many years.

Dr. Yang, Jwing-Ming, for writing the foreword for this book and for his technical advice and publication support. Without Dr. Yang's help, publishing an English book would have been difficult for me. I have learned a lot from him during our recent writing collaboration. I thank him with all my heart for helping me unconditionally.

My grandfather, Liang, Zhi-Xiang, who led me to the introduction of qigong and martial arts. It was his strict discipline that trained me and built a solid foundation for my advancement.

My uncle, Mr. Jeffrey D. S. Liang, and my aunt, Eva, for adopting me when I was a child. Without them, I would not be where I am today. Though political turmoil in China had separated us for nearly forty years, through their effort, I was able to reunite with them in 1981 in Seattle. They later assisted me in gaining employment at the University of British Columbia (UBC), which made it possible for me to immigrate to Canada. It has since changed my whole life. Uncle Jeffrey, once a diplomat, an engineer, and then a cultural and social advocate, has been for years recorded as a biographee in *Marquis Who's Who in the World* and several other Marquis publications. Aunt Eva gained recognition in her teens as a silver medalist in a wushu fighting competition at Chongqing.

My parents, for tirelessly raising me during a time of persecution and turbulence in China, for their continual encouragement to go forward, and for increasing my will to succeed.

My wife, for working so hard to keep our family together and for supporting my work.

Mr. Harry Fan, for offering me my first job in Canada at the Villa Cathy Care Home during a critical time. It gave me an opportunity to make myself known to Canadian communities and to offer my knowledge to the North American people.

Mr. Raymond Ching and Ms. Taisung Wang, for helping to promote Chinese culture at the UBC, for assisting me in receiving my immigration visa to Canada, and for helping me clear difficult problems during a critical time.

Mr. Arthur J. Lee and Dr. W. Robert Morford, for their important help during a critical time. They assisted me in gaining employment at the UBC and immigrating to Canada.

Ms. Sonya Lumhoist-Smith and Dr. Robert Schutz, for continuing to support me in the promotion of Chinese martial arts at the UBC.

Mr. Paul Ha, for his continuous promotion of Chinese martial arts at the university, and for his continuous support and advice on my career.

Mr. Bill Chen, Mr. L. H. Kwan, Mr. Solen Wong, Dr. James Hii, Mr. Michael Levenston, and friends, for giving me their great help.

My friends at the North American Tai Chi Society in Vancouver, the masters and instructors of the International Wushu San So Do, Yang's Martial Arts Association, and SYL Wushu Institute, for their support. Thanks, also, to the friends and students I have met during my travels through China, North America, Canada, and Europe.

Very special thanks to the elder-generation masters, responsible for compiling the 24 and 48 Posture Taijiquan.

It is a great pleasure to work with Mr. Wu, Wen-Ching in completing this book. Wen-Ching is humble, fond of learning, scholarly, morally upright, enthusiastic, and has a high sense of honor and loyalty. He was the 1990 United States National Chinese Martial Arts Competition Grand Champion in both external styles and internal styles. He is a highly accomplished young martial artist, both in taijiquan and kung fu. He has put a lot of time into completing this book. I thank him for the tremendous amount of help he has given me. Also, thanks to all the people who assisted in making this book possible, especially to Reza Farman-Farmaian, for his excellent photography, and Denise Breiter, for her precise editing.

Master Liang, Shou-Yu

Preface by Master Liang, Shou-Yu
(Revised Edition, 1995)

Taijiquan (tai chi chuan) has had more than three hundred years of history in China and has become very popular around the world today. More and more people are getting involved in taijiquan training.

There are five traditional taijiquan styles in China. They are Chen, Yang, Wu, Wǔ, and Sun. However, the most popular is Yang Style. From Yang Style are derived more styles, such as Zheng Zi Taiji and Fu Style Taiji. It is not surprising that there are so many styles of taijiquan. Even everywhere in China, Yang Style Taiji practitioners have different understandings of the sequences. Consequently, the training methods are also different. It is the same for other styles, each of which has different ways of training and different characteristics, depending on the locations in China. From varied research and development, different taijiquan sequences were created. A conservative estimate counts more than thirty different taijiquan sequences.

During the 1950s, the Chinese Athletic Committee, organized a team to compile the 24 Postures of Simplified Taijiquan. This compilation was based on the foundation of Yang Style Taijiquan. The movements of this new simplified taijiquan are easy to learn and the postures are accurate and standardized. Therefore, some people have called it Standardized Taijiquan. These 24 Postures of Simplified Taijiquan have been popularly welcomed and practiced both in China and foreign countries in the last forty years.

I have been teaching 24 Posture Taijiquan since early the 1960s. Based on my last thirty-five years of experience, I feel that this sequence is simple and easy to learn, and is suitable for both men and women of many ages. It has also brought to all of the practitioners the great benefit of health and is, therefore, worthwhile for me to popularize it. In addition, to a taijiquan beginner, this sequence can also be used to build a solid foundation for further study of other styles of taijiquan. To help the reader understand the meaning of each movement in the sequence, I will also introduce the martial applications of each movement. This is the first time the martial applications of 24 Postures will be introduced to the public, both in China and foreign countries. This unique aspect of the book shows that taijiquan is not just dancing or moving exercises.

During the 1970s, the Chinese Athletic Committee compiled the 48 Postures of Taijiquan, which combined the characteristics of Yang, Wu, and Chen Styles. This enables a practitioner to taste the differences of these three styles. This new 48 Postures sequence again has been welcomed by taijiquan practitioners. After you have learned and practiced 24 Posture Taijiquan, if you can practice this 48 Posture Taijiquan, you will enter a new sensational domain of taiji feeling, and therefore generate more interest and deeper understanding.

Master Liang, Shou-Yu
September 7, 1995

CHAPTER ONE

General Introduction

1.1: **Introduction**

Taijiquan (tai chi chuan) is a healing/martial art that combines martial arts movements with energy (*qi* or *chi*) circulation, breathing, and stretching techniques. It utilizes the ancient philosophy of *yin* and *yang* and the five element theories, for its foundation and to establish its training principles. The training of taijiquan includes the integration of mind, qi, and body. The focus on qi circulation was initially used for the purpose of increasing the internal strength of the physical body for combat. The same techniques that were capable of developing internal power for combat also proved to be effective as life-prolonging, healing, and rejuvenating exercises. These health benefits are the primary contributions that led to the popularity of taijiquan today.

In today's hectic life, many of us are often too busy to be concerned about our health, until our health becomes a problem. Lucky for us, modern medicine has a cure for many common diseases. Unfortunately, some are still incurable. Many times the root of the sickness is not corrected, and the sickness reoccurs or manifests itself in other forms. The value of taijiquan is in its potential to strengthen and repair the physical and energetic body, which in turn has the potential to prevent and cure diseases.

With regular practice of taijiquan, it is possible to keep blood and energy circulation smooth in the entire body, and prevent disease. Traditional Chinese medical theory places prevention in the highest esteem, correcting a problem before any symptom occurs. If a problem already exists, it can be regulated through the regular practice of taijiquan, before it causes any major damage. If the problem is already causing damage, then drastic measures may need to be taken to repair it. Once the damage is repaired, the non-jarring, slow, and integrated movements of taijiquan make an excellent recovery exercise for regaining health.

There is a story about a famous Chinese doctor who was greeted with gifts by his grateful patients and was named the greatest doctor of his time. He humbly refused to accept the title. He then told the story about his two older brothers, who were also doctors. Below is a version of the story:

I am the doctor who cures the disease when it has already occurred and is doing damage. My second brother is the doctor who cures the disease when it just starts to occur. My oldest brother is the doctor who prevents disease. My ability to repair physical damage is easily noticeable, and the word of my ability has spread far throughout the country. My second brother's ability to cure the disease before it does any major damage is less noticeable. He is, therefore, only known around this region. My oldest brother's ability to help prevent disease before it occurs is hardly noticeable. He is, therefore, hardly known in his province.

Dear friends, even though I am the most famous of my three brothers, I am not the greatest doctor because I can only repair the damage. My second brother, even though he is less famous than I am, is far greater than I am because he is able to correct the disease before it does any damage. My oldest brother, the least known, is the greatest of us all because he is able to prevent problems before they occur.

So, what is it in taijiquan that gives it this "magical" power? Physically, the slow and relaxed condensing and expanding movements provide a total body exercise. As the muscles are allowed to relax, blood circulation can be improved. This total body exercise is not limited to the arms and legs. It also refers to the ribs, spine, and internal organs. The gentle movements loosen up the spine and ribs, as well as the organs. By "massaging" the organs, you can loosen up the tension around them and increase the blood circulation. Many life-threatening diseases occur from problems associated with the organs, so why not "massage" the organs and keep them healthy? The slow movements allow the body to move with less tension than high-paced movements, which require fast muscle contractions. The slow movements of taijiquan allow the lungs to be more relaxed and to increase the intake of oxygen.

Taijiquan helps release tension created by a hard day at work. Mentally and energetically, tension is released from the head and other areas, where energy stagnates. Modern science has documented that each section of the brain does a specialized set of tasks. Over the course of a day, week, month, or year, we may be overstimulating one section or another of our brain. This overstimulation often creates excess tension that is unable to dissipate from the head. When this happens, we may not be able to think as clearly. We may lose our temper easily or even get headaches. Taijiquan exercise helps to redistribute energy in our bodies by leading excess energy from tense areas, so as to regain balance. Performing taijiquan early in the morning clears the mind and prepares one to tackle any task during the day. That is one of the reasons, to the amazement of many foreign visitors in China, that millions of Chinese practice taijiquan in the park every morning before work. After all, what is disease (dis-ease) but a lack of ease? By learning to live with ease, one prevents disease.

1.2: **The Theoretical Foundation of Taijiquan**

A good understanding of the cultural and historical background of an art can help provide a deeper appreciation of the art. This is especially true for taijiquan. Like all other Chinese arts and science, Chinese culture, as a whole, is the root and foundation of its developments. Chinese view the universe as one interrelated organism, not as separate entities; everything resonates to reach balance and harmony. This view, on a smaller scale, also applies to the human body. It is believed that studying the universe will give us an understanding of the small universe—the human body. Conversely, by studying the small universe, we can gain insight into the cosmos. The Chinese believe that heaven and humans combine as one (*tian ren he yi*). They also believe the human body is a small heaven and earth (small universe), and the universe is a big human body (*yi shen yi xiao ti an di,* [and] *ti an di yi da ren shen*). In this section we will give a brief overview of the yin and yang and five element (*wuxing*) theories of the universe and the concept of energy (qi), and how this applies to the human body—the small universe.

Yin and Yang and Five Element Theories of the Universe

The yin and yang and five element theories are the core of ancient Chinese philosophy. The yin and yang theory is based on the thought that everything in the universe is produced, developed, and constantly changing due to the interaction of yin and yang. The five elements (wuxing) are categories of material things that make up the universe. Wuxing is often translated as five elements, five phases, five processes, five shapes, or five states. The most common translation is five elements. This theory classifies everything into five categories represented by five elements: metal, water, wood, fire, and earth. It explains the interactions among the five elements. It also explains the manifested properties of material things as they undergo changes.

Yin and Yang Theory

Ancient Chinese philosophers believed that everything in the universe was interrelated. Everything in the universe has an opposing yet inseparable counterpart. The counterparts are referred to as yin and yang. Yin and yang is constantly changing. This is the reason for all activity in the universe. This concept of constant change became an approach to understand the laws of nature. The basic theory of yin and yang can be summed up briefly as yin and yang opposition (*yin yang dui li*), yin and yang interdependence (*yin yang hugen*), yin and yang decreasing and increasing (*yin yang xiao zhang*), and yin and yang transformation (*yin yang zhuan hua*).

Yin and yang opposition explains that within all things in nature, there are opposing but coexisting characteristics of yin and yang. For example, the sky is yang and the earth is yin; man is yang and woman is yin; fire is yang and water is yin. However, keep in mind that the terms yin and yang are abstract and relative, not absolute. Under specific conditions, the yin and yang characteristics may change and within the yin or yang, there are subdivisions of yin and yang.

Yin and yang interdependence refers to the interdependent characteristic of yin and yang. One cannot exist without the other. In distinguishing the characteristics of yin and yang, there needs to be a reference. This reference is the yin or yang counterpart. For example, when classifying a cup, the inside is yin and the outside is yang. If the cup doesn't have an outside (yang), it would not be a cup and therefore would not have an inside (yin). All yin and yang must coexist and depend on each other. Without one, there isn't the other.

Yin and yang decreasing and increasing describes the interaction and potential exchange between yin and yang. The existence of yin and yang is not a static state. It is always changing, interchanging potentials. It is always either yin decreasing and yang increasing or yin increasing and yang decreasing. For example, during a twenty-four-hour period, the sun comes up on the horizon (an increase in yang) and evening diminishes it (a decrease in yang). In the afternoon, the sun begins to go down on the horizon, causing a decrease in yang, and as evening approaches, there is an increase in yin. Another example can be seen in the waxing and waning of the moon. This is true for everything in the universe.

Yin and yang transformation describes the way yin and yang properties change into each other. The transformation occurs under extreme conditions of yin and yang decreasing and increasing. For example, if you were to throw a ball straight up, the upward velocity is classified as yang. This speed slows down as it reaches its maximum height (decreasing yang). At the maximum height, the velocity becomes zero (extreme condition), and the ball begins to fall (yang velocity becomes yin velocity).

There is no conclusive evidence on when and how the yin and yang philosophy was first introduced to the Chinese culture. Some say it is at least five thousand years old. Some recent archaeological findings suggest the yin and yang concept may be over ten thousand years old, which is from the discovery of ancient clay pots with markings that may represent yin and yang. This concept was explained in detail during the Zhou dynasty (1122–249 BC) when the Zhou dynasty's *Book of Changes* (*Zhouyi*) was compiled. The contents of *Zhouyi* consist of two volumes. The first is the *Book of Changes* (*Yi Jing* or *I Ching*), which is about prediction and probability. The second volume, *Yi Chuan*, contains the theoretical and philosophical explanation of the *Book of Changes* (*Yi Jing*). *Zhouyi* is the oldest and most influential book of the Chinese classics, containing information about everything from astrology, meteorology, and geology to human relationships. It uses the yin and yang concept to explain the rules of the universe and to analyze everything in it.

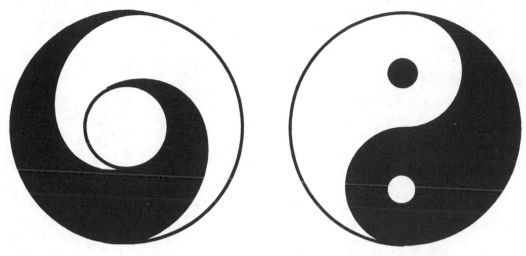

Taiji symbol 1.

Taiji symbol 2.

In the thousands of years since the yin and yang theory was formulated, many symbols have been designed to graphically represent the interrelationship of yin and yang. These symbols representing yin and yang are called *taiji* symbols, from which taijiquan derived its name. Taiji symbol 1 and taiji symbol 2 are just two examples of these symbols. The most commonly used symbol is taiji symbol 2. It has a big circle on the outside, which symbolizes the whole universe. The curvature within the circle symbolizes the opposing yet interdependent nature of yin and yang. The black (yin) and the white (yang) teardrop shapes symbolize the decreasing and increasing as well as the transformation of yin and yang. Within the largest white surface area of the circle is a small black circle. This smaller circle symbolizes the inherent yin (black dot) in yang. Similarly, within the largest black surface of the circle is a small white circle symbolizing the inherent yang in yin. These small circles symbolize that yin and yang are not absolute; there are subdivisions of yin and yang both within yin and within yang.

Five Element (Wuxing) Theory

Ancient philosophers believed that the universe was made up of five fundamental elements: metal, water, wood, fire, and earth. They categorized and associated material things under each of the elements by similarity, kind, and relationship. They called the interactions of the elements, wuxing. "Wu" literally means five, and "xing" literally means behavior, conduct, or to travel. Even though the xing does not have the meaning of elements, it is implied by the five classifications: metal, water, wood, fire, and earth. As these five elements interact with each other, they create the universe as we know it.

Five Elements	Nature				Human Body			
	Seasons	Colors	Directions	Tastes	Yin Organs	Yang Organs	Emotions	Facial Features
Metal	Autumn	White	West	Pungent	Lungs	Large Intestine	Sorrow	Nose
Water	Winter	Black	North	Salty	Kidneys	Bladder	Fear	Ears
Wood	Spring	Green	East	Sour	Liver	Gall Bladder	Anger	Eyes
Fire	Summer	Red	South	Bitter	Heart	Small Intestine	Joy	Tongue
Earth	Late Summer	Yellow	Center	Sweet	Spleen	Stomach	Pensiveness	Mouth

Some correlations of the five elements.

The basic theory behind the five elements can be summed up by two types of cyclic interactions and three types of adverse interactions. The cyclic interactions are mutual nourishment (*xiang sheng*) and mutual restraint (*xiang ke*). The adverse interactions are mutual overrestraint (*xiang cheng*), mutual reverse restraint (*xiang wu*), and mutual burdening (*zi mu xiang ji*).

Mutual nourishment refers to the cyclic enhancement of, or the ability to promote each other, either directly or indirectly. In this cycle, each element both gives and receives nourishment. For example, the wood (tree) element "grows" when it is nourished by the

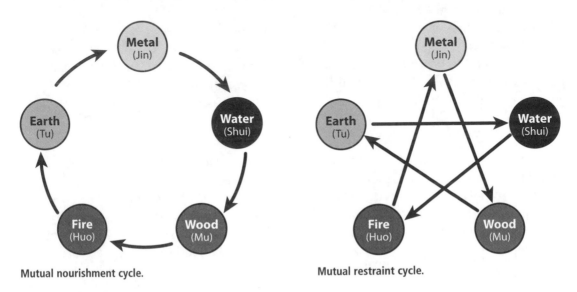

Mutual nourishment cycle.

Mutual restraint cycle.

flow of water. Wood in turn gives nourishment to fire and enhances fire. This exchange of nourishment continues to the next elements until the cycle is completed. This mutual nourishment cycle is also called the "mother and son" relationship.

Mutual restraint refers to the cyclic neutralizing of the elements in order to keep each element in check. In the restraining relationship, each element is capable of restraining the next one and may also be restrained by the previous one. For example, water is capable of putting out fire, fire can melt metal, metal can chop wood, wood (ancient farm tools) can dig up earth, and earth can absorb water. This mutual restraining cycle is also known as a "win-lose relationship."

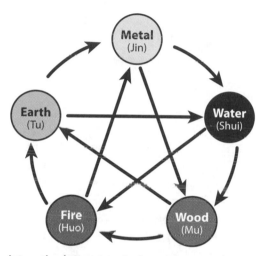

Interaction between mutual nourishment and mutual restraint cycles.

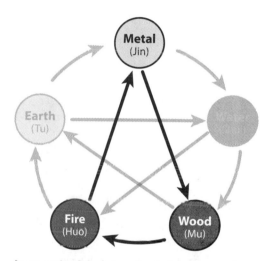

An example of the interaction between mutual nourishment and mutual restraint cycles.

Mutual nourishment and mutual restraint are not independent cycles. They interact with each other and are closely related. For example, metal can restrain wood, yet wood is able to nourish fire, which in turn can restrain metal. Initially, this type of reasoning seems to indicate that nothing would exist in this cyclic situation. If all things in the universe were to exist in equal quantities and were equally effective, the elements would in fact inhibit each other and nothing would happen. However, the elements are not present equally and at the same time, which allows this cyclic process to manifest itself. This mutual nourishing and restraining keeps nature in a system of checks and balances.

Mutual overrestraint describes an abnormal condition in the five element cycle. It refers to excessive restraining in the mutual restraint cycle. It is a situation where the element being restrained is too weak or the restraining element is too strong; thus, an unbalanced or adverse effect occurs.

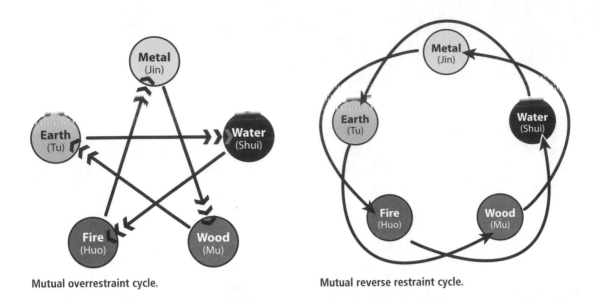

Mutual overrestraint cycle.

Mutual reverse restraint cycle.

Mutual reverse restraint describes another abnormal condition in the five element cycle. It is the reverse of the mutual restraint cycle. In this case, the restraining element is too "weak" or the element being restrained is too "strong"; then a reversal of the mutual restraint cycle occurs.

Mutual burdening is yet another abnormal condition in the five element cycle. It is an adverse condition of the mutual nourishment cycle in which the direction of flow in nourishment is unbalanced or reversed.

Energy (Qi) Concept

The primary attempt of the yin and yang and five element theories is to explain the balance or imbalance of qi. Qi is a Chinese term used to refer to all types of energy. As examples, the weather condition is called heaven's energy (*tian qi*), the energy within the human body is called human energy (*ren qi*), the air we breathe is called air energy (*kong qi*), and the energy required to run an electric motor is called electric energy (*dian qi*). Qi is the intrinsic substance or the vital force behind all things (elements) in the universe.

Qigong (*chi kung*) is a term used to describe the study of qi. It is most often associated with the study of qi in the human body. Keep in mind, however, because we are part of nature, the study of human qi cannot be separated from the study of universal qi. Today, the term qigong is commonly used to describe a set of exercises that helps calm the mind, regulate the breathing, and relax the physical body, which in turn helps lead to health and longevity.

After thousands of years of research and development, many effective and practical qigong techniques have been devised to combat the "evil" influences of nature. These exercises were also created to strengthen the body, to prevent sickness, and to speed recovery. This research helped to confirm that energy (qi), which is not visible to the human eye, can be felt as a warm, tingling sensation and has set pathways in the human body. This energy in the human body, called human energy (ren qi) or simply qi, travels through set pathways called meridians. The meridians consist of the eight extraordinary vessels, twelve channels, and three hundred plus cavities, which connect the different parts of the body. The vessels and channels are the reservoirs and rivers for the transportation of qi. The cavities are the points through which the reservoirs or rivers can be accessed, using acupressure, acupuncture, moxibustion, or massage. These energy meridians must be full and flowing evenly to prevent illness and to remove blockages in the body.

As early as the Shang dynasty (1766–1123 BC), Chinese people used stone probes (*bianshi*) to stimulate the cavities, to relieve pressure and pain, and to balance energy circulation. It was not until the Song dynasty (AD 960–1126) during the reign of Emperor Ren-zong (AD 1023–1059) that an energy diagram was systematically charted. Historical records indicate that in AD 1034, Emperor Ren-zong got seriously ill and was cured by one of his palace doctors, Dr. Xu Xi, who used acupuncture techniques. During Dr. Xu's award ceremony, he asked the emperor to advocate the use of acupuncture and its research. At that time, some acupuncture diagrams were available, but they were not consistent. Many acupuncturists kept their discoveries secret, so there wasn't a standard set for acupuncture. To reduce the inconsistencies and to develop a higher standard for acupuncture, Emperor Ren-zong ordered Dr. Wang, Wei-yi to accurately chart the acupuncture points in the human body and to build two bronze men with the points clearly marked.

Modern versions of acupuncture charts are derivatives of Dr. Wang's Bronze Man. Today, modern technology has enabled us to locate the points with electrical instruments. These points are all consistent with Dr. Wang's findings hundreds of years ago. Legend has it that Dr. Wang was able to chart the points with such precision because he was able to experiment on real people. With permission from the emperor, Dr. Wang offered convicted criminals the possibility of freedom or money for their families in exchange for their cooperation with charting the acupuncture points. Dr. Wang proceeded with the experimentation by inserting acupuncture needles and recording sensations or feedback given by the volunteers in order to chart the points accurately.

The Human Body as a Small Universe

The yin and yang theory is primarily about the opposing, interdependent, decreasing and increasing, and transformational nature of material things. The five element theory categorizes material things and uses the natural rhythms that govern them to describe the relationship among them. Since humans are a part of nature and nature contains the "ingredients" essential to human survival, the changes in nature will directly or indirectly affect our bodies. It is obvious that humans and nature are very closely linked. Because of this close tie with nature, the yin and yang and the five element theories also govern the functioning of the human system on a small scale.

The acupuncture meridians provide the transportation of qi among the organs (elements) and maintain the mutual nourishment and mutual restraint cycles in a harmonious relationship. Because the body is viewed as a whole, illness in one part of the body will also manifest itself in other parts. To cure an illness of one organ, Chinese doctors may have to treat other organs because of the cyclic relationship of the organs. To the amazement of many people, Chinese doctors may treat the organ by treating the limbs because the arms and legs contain the qi extensions of the organs.

Chinese medicine believes that sickness is the result of the body's inability to properly adapt and adjust to the "evil" influences of nature. Because humans are a part of nature, any change in nature will inevitably affect the human body. When the "evil" influences of nature go above and beyond human adaptability, an overrestraint condition occurs, and the balance between humans and nature is destroyed. The human body functions will then be affected, and sickness will result. Sickness will last until the body can attain the proper balance. An example of this can be seen during the change of seasons. When weather changes from hot to cold rapidly, people who are not able to make the adjustment smoothly often get colds or the flu. This is especially obvious when an "unseasoned" person from a very warm climate is introduced to an extremely cold climate for the first time. People who are used to the fluctuating weather are usually not affected by it.

Based on the same energy theory, exercise and breathing techniques were created to adjust the imbalance of energy in the body, to build energy, and to increase adaptability to the environment. These exercises are known as *Dao yin* and *tu na*. Dao yin is the art of guiding the qi to achieve harmony, and stretching the body to "massage" the cavities in order to reduce qi stagnation and to attain flexibility (*Dao qi ling he, yin ti lingrou*). Tu na is the art of expelling "old" air and drawing in the "new" air (*tu gu na xin*)—the art of breathing. The combination of Dao yin and tu na techniques, along with the circular movements of martial arts, became the healing martial art known as taijiquan.

1.3: **Taijiquan History**

Creation of Taijiquan

There are many theories concerning the founding of taijiquan. We will briefly discuss three of the major theories. The first theory is that the Daoist (*Taoist*) Zhang,

San-feng in the Northern Song dynasty (AD 960–1126) created taijiquan. The second is that the prolific writer of taijiquan treatises Wang, Zong-yue created taijiquan. The third theory is that Chen, Wang-ting, a military officer in the latter part of the Ming dynasty, created taijiquan.

However, it is known that as early as the fourth century BC, the life-nourishing techniques (*yang shen fa*) were being practiced. They included bending, expanding, condensing, and extending movements, as well as breathing techniques and qi circulation, similar to taijiquan's internal exercises. Publications, such as the *Six Animal Play* (*Liuqinxi*) written by Dr. Lui An (179–122 BC) and the *Five Animal Play* (*Wuqinxi*), rewritten by Dr. Hua Tuo (one of the greatest doctors in Chinese history), integrated breathing techniques with the movements of animals to improve health.

It is also known that in the Liang dynasty (AD 502–557) and in the Tang dynasty (AD 618–907) there were already techniques resembling taijiquan. The only difference was in their names. They were named thirty-seven postures (*san shi qi shi*), post-heaven techniques (*hou tian fa*), and small nine heaven (*xiao jiu tian*). Even though the names were different, the principles were similar.

Zhang, San-feng Theory

The historical records of Zhang, San-feng are not very consistent with one another. According to the Song dynasty records in *Wangzhengnan Muzhiming*, "The Song dynasty's Zhang, San-feng was a Wudang Daoist Monk." *Wangzhengnan Muzhiming* was written in AD 1669 by Huang, Li-zhou, a famous scholar of the Qing dynasty (AD 1644–1912). Huang wrote that during the Song dynasty, Zhang, San-feng dreamed that Emperor Yuan taught him martial arts. There are no other earlier documents that indicate Zhang, San-feng knew any martial arts. Below are some quotes from the *Wangzhengnan Muzhiming*:

> Emperor Hui-zong summoned him. The road to the palace was blocked by robbers, [and] he could not go forward. At night he dreamed that Emperor Yuan taught him martial techniques. At dawn, by himself, he killed a hundred robbers.

According to the Ming dynasty record, *Mingshi Fangjizhuan*,

> Zhang, San-feng of Liaodongyi County was named Quan-yi, or Jun-bao. San-feng was his Daoist name. Because he didn't keep himself clean and neat, he was nicknamed Sloppy Zhang. He was big and tall, had the look of a turtle and a back like a crane, with large ears, round eyes, and a beard as long as a spear tassel. Winter and summer, he wore the same Daoist outfit. He could eat a bushel of food, or not eat for several days or months.

He walked thousands of kilometers a day, loved to have fun, and acted as though there were no one else around him but himself. He often traveled with his disciple to the Wudang Mountains and built grass huts to live in. In the twenty-fourth year of Hongwu (AD 1391), Emperor Ming, Tai-zu heard about Zhang, San-feng and sent messengers to look for him, but without success.

Some records indicate that Zhang was made an immortal figure as the result of the struggle for power in the Ming dynasty. When the first Ming emperor died, the grandson of the emperor, Jian-wen, was made the successor because the crown prince, Jian-wen's father, died at a young age. Emperor Jian-wen's uncle, Yong-le, unhappy with the arrangement, found an excuse to revolt against the young Emperor Jian-wen and took over the throne. Rumor had it that Emperor Jian-wen survived the ordeal. Emperor Yong-le, petrified with the thought that the outcast Emperor Jian-wen might organize a counterrevolution against him, sent assassins to search for him.

Needing an excuse to send out a search party, Emperor Yong-le made up a reason to look for the immortal Zhang, San-feng. For over twenty years, Emperor Yong-le sent assassins all over the empire and overseas searching for Emperor Jian-wen, but without success. When Emperor Yong-le finally stopped his search, the news of the search for the immortal Zhang, San-feng had spread all over the empire. To cover up the real reason for the search and his lies to the people, he commanded that a temple be built in the Wudang Mountains to honor Zhang, San-feng. The construction was believed to include the labor of over three hundred thousand people at a cost of over several million ounces of silver. From then on, Zhang, San-feng of the Wudang Mountain became a legendary figure in Chinese society.

It is also recorded in the *Ming Langying Qixiu Leigao*:

> Immortal Zhang, named Jun-bao, or Quan-yi, was called by the Daoist name Xuan-xuan. He was nicknamed by the laymen as Sloppy Zhang. In the third year of Tianshun (AD 1459), he visited the emperor. A picture was drawn. The picture showed him with a straight beard and a moustache, a tuft at the back of his head, a purple face, a big stomach, and holding a bamboo hat in his hand. At the top of the picture was an honorary inscription by the emperor, honoring Zhang as a knowledgeable and prestigious Daoist.

Other sources said that Zhang, San-feng's techniques came from the Daoist Feng, Yi-yuan. Yet another said that Zhang, San-feng was an ancient Daoist hermit who, after observing a fight between a crane and a snake, was enlightened and invented taijiquan.

Wang, Zong-yue Theory

Wang, Zong-yue's *Taijiquan Classics* are well known by taijiquan practitioners. Wang, Zong-yue systematically summarized the principles of taijiquan, using the yin and yang theory. He was the first to call this martial art taijiquan. He wrote: "What is taiji? It is generated from *wuji*. It is the mother of yin and yang. When it moves, it divides. At rest, it reunites." He was once mistaken to be Wang Zong of the Ming dynasty. This mistake in identity also led some to believe that taijiquan was created by Wang Zong in the Ming dynasty. It also made many believe that Jiang Fa, a military officer in the later part of Ming dynasty, learned from Wang, Zong-yue. This same belief later led many to believe that Jiang Fa taught taijiquan to the Chen family, when he took refuge at Chen Village (Chenjiagou) as a servant. This theory came from an interpretation in the book *Taijiquan Brief* (*Taijiquan Xiaoxu*), written by Li, Yi-yu (AD 1832–1892). In his book, Li, Yi-yu stated that the creator of taijiquan is unknown, but Wang, Zong-yue had described the art in detail. It was believed that Jiang Fa learned from Wang, Zong-yue and then Jiang Fa taught the art to the Chens in Chen Village.

Chen, Wang-ting Theory

Another theory on the creation of taijiquan is the Chen, Wang-ting[1] theory. Chen, Wang-ting (AD ?–1719) was a military officer during the latter part of the Ming dynasty (AD 1368–1644). Some martial arts historians believe that Chen combined the *Martial Classic in Thirty-Two Postures* (*Quanjing Sanshier Shi*)[2] and the *Daoist Yellow Courtyard Classic* (*Huangtingjing*) with his personal martial background and created taijiquan. Chen received many honors for his bravery and accomplishments during the end of the Ming dynasty. When the Ming dynasty was defeated and the Qing dynasty came into power (AD 1644–1912), he became a hermit and spent time teaching martial arts to his relatives and "creating fists" when he wasn't farming. In the *History of the Chen Family* it stated next to Chen, Wang-ting's name, "Wang-ting, also known as Zou-ting, was a martial artist during the end of the Ming dynasty and a scholar during the beginning of the Qing dynasty. Well-known for his *wushu* (martial arts) in Shandong Province, [he] was the founder of Chen Family Martial Arts. He defeated over one thousand bandits. He was a born hero."

Taijiquan Developments after the Chen Family

The Chen family passed down its lineage until the fourteenth generation of Chens in Chen Village. Then it was subdivided into Old Frame Style and New Frame Style. The New Frame Style was created by Chen, You-ben. The Old Frame Style was continued by Chen, Chang-xing. Chen, Chang-xing, aside from passing down the art to his son, Geng-yun, and his relatives, Chen, Huai-yuan and Chen, Hua-mei, also taught

Yang, Lu-chan (AD 1799–1872) and Li, Bo-kui. Chen, Chang-xing's lineage was called Thirteen Posture Old Frame.

Later, Yang, Lu-chan passed the art to two of his sons, Yang, Ban-hou (AD 1837–1892) and Yang, Jian-hou (AD 1839–1917). Then, Jian-hou passed the art to his sons, Shao-hou (AD 1862–1930) and Cheng-fu (AD 1883–1936), and to his disciples. Shao-hou and Cheng-fu continued to pass down the art to their sons and disciples. This became what is commonly called the Yang Style. Besides the Yang Style, Chen, Qing-ping (AD 1795–1868) learned Chen, You-ben's New Frame Style and began the *Zhaobao* Style. Wǔ, Yu-xiang (AD 1812–1880) learned from Yang, Lu-chan and Chen, Qing-ping, and created Wǔ Style. Li, Yi-yu (AD 1832–1892) learned the art from the Wǔ Style. He, Wei-zhen (AD 1849–920) learned from Li, Yi-yu and taught it to Sun, Lu-tang (AD 1861–1932). Sun, Lu-tang's lineage is known as Sun Style today.

Wu Style is another very popular style of taijiquan now practiced in China. Wu Style derived from Yang Style. Yang, Ban-hou, son of Yang, Lu-chan, taught a modified Small Frame Yang Style to Wu, Quan-you (AD 1834–1902). Wu, Quan-you taught his son, Wu, Jian-quan (AD 1870–1942). Wu, Jian-quan popularized the Small Frame Yang Style. Wu, Jian-quan's taijiquan is now known as Wu Style Taijiquan. After Wu, Jian-quan died, his sons, Wu, Gong-yi and Wu, Gong-zao, and his daughter, Wu, Ying-hua, carried on their father's legacy and popularized Wu Style Taijiquan.

In 1956, the Simplified Taijiquan (or 24 Posture Taijiquan which is the primary focus of this book) was compiled. In 1976, another sequence was compiled. It was called 48 Posture Taijiquan. Tremendous efforts were put into promoting the 24 Posture Taijiquan, which was derived from the traditional Yang Style Taijiquan long form. It was the result of many taijiquan masters working toward standardizing and simplifying taijiquan for use as a health-promoting exercise. Many of the more complicated and repeated movements were deleted from the long form for ease of learning and practicing. The sequence starts off with very simple movements and gradually becomes more complicated. It has both left and right sides for many of the postures, in contrast to the traditional long form. Even though the 24 Posture Taijiquan sequence is a simplified version of the long form, it is still a traditional sequence with the original martial applications in every movement.

1.4: **Brief History of the Yang Family**

The 24 Posture Taijiquan sequence is based on the traditional Yang Style long form. Therefore, it may be of interest to readers to read some exciting stories about the founder of Yang Style and his descendants. Most of the information below is translated from the book *Taijiquan, Saber, Sword, Staff, and Sparring*, by Chen, Yan-lin. Please see the bibliography for book details.

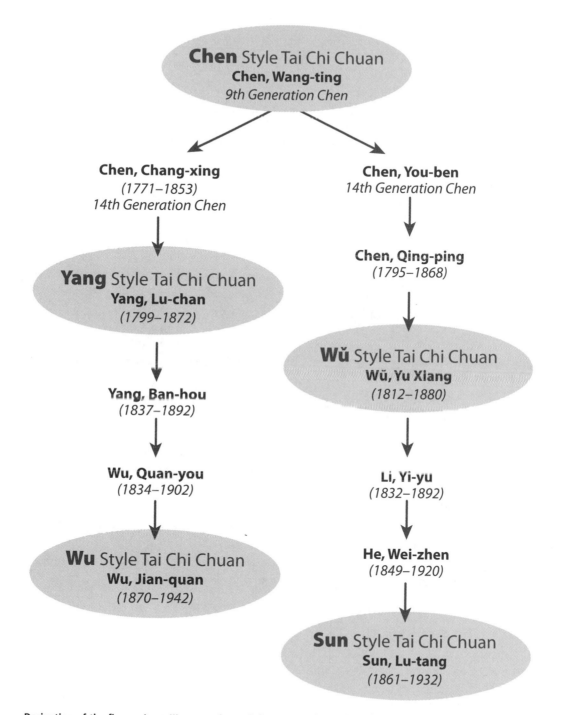

Chen Style Tai Chi Chuan
Chen, Wang-ting
9th Generation Chen

Chen, Chang-xing
(1771–1853)
14th Generation Chen

Chen, You-ben
14th Generation Chen

Chen, Qing-ping
(1795–1868)

Yang Style Tai Chi Chuan
Yang, Lu-chan
(1799–1872)

Wŭ Style Tai Chi Chuan
Wŭ, Yu Xiang
(1812–1880)

Yang, Ban-hou
(1837–1892)

Wu, Quan-you
(1834–1902)

Li, Yi-yu
(1832–1892)

He, Wei-zhen
(1849–1920)

Wu Style Tai Chi Chuan
Wu, Jian-quan
(1870–1942)

Sun Style Tai Chi Chuan
Sun, Lu-tang
(1861–1932)

Derivation of the five major taijiquan styles and the names of their founders.

Yang, Lu-chan

Yang, Fu-kui, also known as Yang, Lu-chan, was a native of Yongnianxian, Guang-ping County, Hebei Province. He was born in the fourth year of Jiaqing, the eleventh year of Tongzhi (AD 1799). When he was young, he went to Chen Village in Henan to study taijiquan from Chen, Chang-xing. At that time, those who learned from the Chens were mostly Chen relatives. Outsiders were seldom allowed to practice with them. Yang, an outsider, was no exception. But because his heart was set on learning, he never gave up. Yang stayed at Chen Village for several years without learning anything. One night, Yang woke up and heard "heng" and "ha" sounds in the adjacent yard. He got up and traced the phenomenon to a compound with several buildings. He peeked through a crack in the wall. There he saw his master teaching a few disciples the techniques of grasping and controlling, and emitting power. Dumfounded by the techniques, he went to watch the practice sessions every night. After every observation, he immediately went back to his room to ponder and study what he observed. Because of this, his martial arts skills improved significantly. One day, Chen ordered Yang to spar with the other disciples. All the disciples lost to Yang. Chen, Chang-xing was surprised and realized Yang's talent. He then began to teach Yang the complete secrets of the art.

After Yang returned to his hometown, he began to teach and pass down his knowledge to the townspeople. There were many who studied from him. The techniques taught by Yang were called the Neutralizing Style or Soft Style because the movements were soft and could neutralize the opponent's power. Later, Yang went to Beijing. There were many royal family members and officers who learned from him. Yang was appointed by the Qing's military as a martial arts teacher.

Yang was a hardheaded person and loved to compare and try his techniques against other styles of martial arts. He often carried a spear and a small bag as he traveled around the Northern provinces. Wherever he went, he would challenge local well-known martial artists. Whenever he heard of anyone claiming to be unmatched by anyone else, he would insist and force the person to a challenge. He never hurt anyone in his challenges. Because his skill was at such a high level, he was undefeated in all his matches. Therefore, he was nicknamed Undefeatable Yang. There were many interesting stories about Yang's life. Here are a few selected ones:

1. When Yang was at Guangping, he often fought with people on the castle wall. One opponent was unable to defend against Yang's attacks and kept on retreating to the edge of the wall. Yang's opponent, unable to keep his balance began to fall over the edge. At the instant before the opponent fell, Yang, from about thirty feet away, leaped forward, caught the opponent's foot, and saved him from falling to his death.

2.   Yang was exceptionally good at using the spear. Any light object that made contact with his spear would be tossed away. Yang's way of putting out a fire was to move sections of the wall with his spear, so that the fire would not spread. He was also capable of throwing arrows to his target while on horseback without using a bow. Not once in a hundred throws would he miss his target.

3.   On yet another day, Yang was fishing at a lake. Two other martial artists were passing behind Yang. Because of Yang's high reputation, they dared not challenge him. They saw Yang facing the lake fishing and thought of taking advantage of this opportunity. They plotted to push Yang in the water and ruin his reputation. They approached Yang until they were a few steps away; then they rushed forward and attacked him. Yang had already sensed the attackers' intention. Just as the two attackers' hands reached his back, he arched his chest and rounded his back, and executed the high pat on horse technique. As his back arched and head bowed, the two attackers were bounced into the water simultaneously. He then said to them that he would be easy on them today, but if they were on the ground, he would have punished them more severely. The two attackers quickly swam away.

4.   When Yang was visiting Beijing, a famous martial arts teacher heard about his nickname, Undefeatable Yang, and was very envious and eager to challenge him. Yang politely refused at first. The teacher thought Yang was afraid and insisted. Unable to refuse, Yang finally accepted. He laughed and told the teacher since he was so insistent on the challenge, he should first punch Yang three times. The teacher gladly agreed. He raised his fist and struck Yang's stomach with all his might. Yang laughed and uttered the "ha" sound. Before the end of the resonating ha sound, the challenger fell face first thirty feet away.

Yang, Lu-chan's Sons

Yang, Lu-chan had three sons. The oldest son, who was named Yang Qi, died at an early age. The second son was named Yang Yu. The third son was named Yang Jian. Both sons were capable of carrying on their father's art.

Yang Yu, popularly known as Yang, Ban-hou, was often called Mr. Second Son. He was born in the seventeenth year of Daoguang (AD 1837). He began studying taijiquan with his father at a young age. He studied hard every day, no matter how hot or cold the weather was. His father never allowed him any break. He was often scolded and whipped by his father, and had to run for his life a few times. He was a hardheaded person, good in free fighting, and loved to emit power onto others. Oftentimes, when he struck his opponents, red marks would appear on their bodies. The opponents being hit often fell back over thirty feet. When Yang, Ban-hou was young, he fought with a strong and powerful teacher from another martial arts style. He grabbed Yang, Ban-hou's wrist and did not allow him to neutralize. Yang, Ban-hou then emitted power (cold *jin*). His opponent could not hold on and was bounced away. Yang, Ban-hou was so proud of himself that he went home and told his father about the incident. His father heard the story, laughed, and said, "Winning is joyous, but too bad you tore your sleeve. The power you emitted was not real taijiquan power." Yang Yu looked at his sleeve and saw that it was really torn and left with disappointment. After that incident, he practiced harder and harder until he became a superb martial artist.

Yang, Ban-hou modified the Small Frame Yang Style and taught it to a Manchurian named Wu, Quan-you. Wu, Quan-you passed the art to his son, Wu, Jian-quan. Wu, Jian-quan's taijiquan became known as today's Wu Style.

Yang Jian was also known as Yang, Jian-hou or Yang, Jing-hu. In his later years, he was also called Mr. Old Man. He was born in the twenty-second year of Daoguang (AD 1842). He also started his training at a young age. His father was strict and hard on him, and watched him practice daily, not allowing him to slack off. His body and mind were worked to the limits. On several occasions, he almost died of exhaustion. Fortunately, he was rescued before it was too late.

His personality was gentler than his brother's. There were many who studied from him. He taught Large, Medium, and Small Frame Styles. His ability included the coordination of hard and soft power. At that time, the people who studied from him were martial artists who were good with both saber and sword. When they sparred, Yang, Jian-hou needed only to use a dust brush to defeat them. Every time his brush touched the student's wrist, he controlled the student. The student would become defensive and unable to get close enough to strike him. He was also good with the use of spear and staff. He could emit any type of power to the tip of the stick. When another's stick would come in contact with his, it would always bounce back with the other person. His whole body could emit power. The instant he released the "ha" sound, power (jin) was emitted. He was also good at throwing darts. He could hit his target every time. With three or four darts in hand, he could often shoot at three or four flying birds at once.

Yang, Jian-hou's most amazing feat was his ability to retain a sparrow on his hand without allowing it to fly away. The reason is that before birds take off, they need to push down with their feet; the rebound allows them to take off. Yang, Jian-hou was able to feel the bird's feet sinking and softly neutralized the push. The sparrow, unable to create enough force to rebound, was unable to take off. From this it was obvious that his sensitivity was so superb and amazing that no one could hope to match it.

In his later years, Yang, Jian-hou slept with his clothes on so he could get up quickly and practice. His servants often heard resonating sounds from his bedroom. In the sixth year of the Republic (AD 1917) he died of natural causes. A few hours before his death, he had a dream about his death. He called on his disciples and three sons to give them his will. He bathed and changed clothes. Then he died with a smile on his face.

Yang, Lu-chan's Grandsons

Yang, Lu-chan's third son, Yang, Jian-hou, had three sons. His eldest son was named Yang, Zhao-xiong, his second son was named Yang, Zhao-yuan but died at a young age, and his third son was named Yang, Zhao-qing.

Yang, Zhao-xiong, also known as Yang, Meng-xiang, and later also known as Yang, Shao-hou, was often called Mr. Oldest. He was born in the first year of Tongzhi (AD 1862). He started to learn taijiquan when he was seven years old. He had a hardheaded personality, loved to emit power on others, was good in sparring, and inherited many of his older uncle's characteristics. He reached a high level of martial arts ability. He was fast and firm in his movements. Every movement had to be close and just right. This was the same in his teaching philosophy. Because he loved to attack in sparring, many students could not endure it. Therefore, he had few students. He had a deep understanding of borrowing jin, cold jin, intercepting jin, and cross space jin. Unfortunately, he did not wish to teach many people. Therefore, few people knew of him. In the eighteenth year of the Republic (AD 1928), he had a son named Yang, Zhen-sheng.

Yang, Zhao-qing, also known as Yang, Cheng-fu, was nicknamed Mr. Third Son. He was born in the ninth year of Guangxu (AD 1883). He had a mild and gentle personality and didn't care much for martial arts when he was young. It was not until his teens that he began learning from his father. When his father was alive, he was not deeply involved with the study and consequently did not really understand the key secrets of the art. After his father died, he realized his mistake and began to practice hard day and night, eventually reaching high prestige. Many of his abilities were the result of his personal research and practice. He was an extremely gifted individual. Had he practiced hard when he was young, he could have been more accomplished than his grandfather. He was strong and big, externally soft as cotton, internally hard as iron. His abilities to lead others' power and emit his own power were of the highest accomplishment. He taught primarily the large postures, asking that the postures be open and extended. This is almost the opposite of his older brother's teaching approach. Because of his gentle nature, he had many followers.

Yang, Cheng-fu was the first taijiquan master willing to openly share his family secrets with the public. In 1926, the Central Guoshu Institute was founded. Yang, Cheng-fu was invited to be the taijiquan teacher, and his name spread all over the country. Today, members of the fourth generation of Yang, Lu-chan, are still teaching their family style. Yang, Zhen-duo (AD 1924), third son of Yang, Cheng-fu, is now teaching taijiquan in Taiyuan City, Shanxi Province. He also travels abroad, sharing his great-grandfather's legacy to taijiquan enthusiasts all over the world.

Endnotes

1.   Historians have proposed that Chen, Wang-ting might be Chen, Yuting because the Chinese character for "Wang" and for "Yu" differ by only one short stroke. Also, the Chinese character for "Wang" was interchangeable with "Yu." It is plausible that "Wang" should have been "Yu." Because no conclusive evidence is available to the authors at this time, "Wang" is used instead of "Yu."

2.   "The Martial Classic in Thirty-Two Postures" is a section of *The New Book of Effective Disciplines (Jixiao Xinshu)* compiled and written by Marshal Qi, Ji-guang. It is a military and martial arts book. "The Martial Classic in Thirty-Two Postures" mentioned the well-known styles of (wushu) martial arts during Marshal Qi's time. Some of the major styles mentioned are Shaolin, Eagle Claw, and Six Step Monkey Fist. There was no mention of taijiquan, indicating that taijiquan was either not created yet or not a well-known style when Marshal Qi wrote his book.

CHAPTER TWO

Guidelines for Taijiquan Practice

2.1: Introduction

To successfully learn taijiquan (tai chi chuan), you will need to understand some of the principles and guidelines that have accumulated over the centuries by masters of this ancient art. These principles and guidelines are the foundation of taijiquan. In this chapter, we will introduce the general theories behind taijiquan, and the guidelines for physical and mental awareness during practice.

To achieve the maximum benefit from taijiquan practice, it is said that you should practice taijiquan twenty-four hours a day. This doesn't mean that you need to do the taijiquan sequence all the time, but you need to make taijiquan a way of life. The practice of taijiquan will not only provide a whole body workout, but it will also cultivate the energy within your body, increase your mental awareness and centering, and build good habits for proper body alignment. When you have accomplished these goals in practice, you will automatically carry these good habits into your daily life. You will gain a greater awareness of yourself, keeping your physical body properly aligned while sitting, standing, driving, eating, watching TV, working, typing, brushing your teeth, and everything else you do regularly. This is what is meant by practicing taijiquan twenty-four hours a day and making taijiquan a way of life.

2.2: Guidelines for Body Movements

The guidelines in this section are not only used for performing taijiquan as a health exercise, but are also used for martial arts. We will briefly explain the martial arts applications. We will also introduce some of the important guidelines related to each section of the body.

1. Head: Vitality of Spirit Leads to the Top of the Head (Xu Ling Ding Jin)

"Vitality of spirit leads to the top of the head" implies the energizing of your head by a slight lifted feeling. When your head is slightly lifted, it will be upright, with the neck relaxed, and you will appear to have a sense of vitality. With your head upright, it will be easier to keep your balance. To have a suspended feeling, imagine that the *baihui* cavity on top of your head is being suspended by a thread.

2.   Eyes: Eyes Focus with Concentration (Yan Shen Zhu Shi)

Your eyes are generally the first to move when you generate intent with your mind. When practicing taijiquan for health, your eyes correspond with the arm or leg performing the most important movement at the time. When your eyes are focused in the direction of your primary limb, you express the intent of the movement. This way your movements are alive, have a pleasing, artistic appeal, and express the vitality of your spirit.

Today, taijiquan is primarily used as a healing exercise. The focus of your eyes corresponds to your mind, leading the movement of qi (chi). For example, if you were to pick up a pencil from the floor, your eyes usually look in the direction of the pencil first, ahead of your movement. Your hand then proceeds to pick up the pencil, thus showing that the qi led to the hand by your mind caused the action of picking up the pencil. In this type of focusing, the eyes focus on the movement of the primary limb. On the other hand, the martial arts focus is quite different—it is primarily to show a sense of enemy and to raise the vitality of your spirit. In applying the posture as a martial technique, your eyes should focus in the direction of your opponent, not the movement of your limbs.

3.   Mouth: Tongue Gently Touches the Roof of the Mouth (She Qing Ding Shan Ge)

After a hard day, you may find yourself with your teeth clenched unintentionally. Any tension in the mouth can restrict your breathing. Pay attention to your jaw, making sure it is not tensed. During practice, keep your mouth closed, with your lips lightly touching each other. Then touch the tip of your tongue to the roof of your mouth. With your tongue touching the roof of your mouth, saliva will be generated. Your saliva is not only an excellent digestive juice, but it is also an excellent "moisturizer" and "coolant" for your body during taijiquan practice.

Energetically, your tongue connects the conception vessel and the governing vessel. The conception vessel has its primary energy path from your mouth down along the centerline of your throat, chest, and abdomen to your perineum area. The governing vessel has its primary energy path from your perineum up along the midline of your spine to your neck, and it loops over your head to your mouth. Your tongue serves as a bridge to connect the two vessels, providing a complete circuit for a smooth energy transition between the two vessels.

4. Torso: Body Centered and Upright (Shen Ti Zhong Zheng)

Unnecessary tension in your muscles and joints is generated when your body leans or twists excessively. Over the years, certain work conditions may help develop habits that put your body under undue stress, due to improper alignment. All these misalignments need to be corrected before permanent damage occurs. This guideline sets the criteria for proper torso alignment. It allows the body to be relaxed, prevents undue tension, and improves smooth circulation for blood and qi.

The human spine has three natural curves: one at the cervical vertebrae, one at the thoracic vertebrae, and one at the lumbar vertebrae. Keeping the body centered and upright implies that the torso be naturally upright. It doesn't mean the spine should be completely straight, which in reality is not possible. To prevent your body from leaning, it is necessary to tuck your sacrum in slightly. By tucking in your sacrum, you can lessen the stress on your lower back and allow your waist to move more freely. The guideline, sacrum centered and upright (*weilu zhong zheng*), is often used in conjunction with the guideline, body centered and upright. Of course, if your head is not upright, your torso will be affected. Therefore, the guideline, vitality of spirit leads to the top of the head, must also be followed to keep the body centered and upright.

5. Chest and Back: Arc Your Chest and Round Your Back (Han Xiong Ba Bei)

With your chest naturally relaxed and arced in slightly, reducing the pressure on your lungs, you allow deeper and more relaxed breathing. The slight movements of your chest provide direct stimulation and exercise to your organs. It is like a gentle massage, loosening up whatever stagnation there may be in the fasciae layers surrounding your organs. The slight arcing of your chest makes the back slightly rounded with a slightly lifted feeling. When training taijiquan as a fighting art, the chest is arced in farther with the back more rounded. The reason for this is to create the potential for power release. It is like a bow being pulled, storing the potential to release an arrow.

6. Waist and Hips: Loosen Your Waist and Hips (Song Yao Song Kua)

The 206 bones in our bodies are "threaded" together for weight bearing and for a variety of movements. The waist, which connects your upper body and lower body, has a significant influence on the movements of the entire body. Through the connecting ligaments, once the waist moves, the other joints in the body are affected.

Located around your waist area are your *dan tian* and your kidneys. According to Chinese acupuncture, residing in the kidneys is one of the original essences (*yuan jing*). By exercising your waist, you will be stimulating the kidneys—keeping them healthy and functioning properly. It is said by the Chinese that with strong kidneys, your original essence will be sufficient, your qi will be abundant, your spirit will be clear, and your eyes will be bright.

From a martial arts standpoint, the waist is capable of increasing your power and the speed of your techniques. When your waist is loose, the power generated by your legs can easily be transmitted to your arms. Adding the power that can be generated by your waist, your martial potential will be highly improved. On the other hand, if your waist is stiff, then power from your legs will be restricted by your waist, lessening your power manifestation. According to taijiquan theory, the root is at your feet; power is generated by your legs and directed by your waist, and then expressed through your fingers. To adhere to this principle, your upper body must be upright and your stance must be comfortable.

7.   Arms and Shoulders: Sink the Shoulders and Drop the Elbows (Chen Jian Chui Zhou)

Sink the shoulders (*chen jian*) requires that the shoulder joints be loose. Let your arms hang down naturally. Drop the elbows (*chui zhou*) implies the lowering of your elbows. People involved in stress-related work often find themselves with their shoulders raised. When this happens, the lungs are constricted from the tension caused by the shoulders. This will restrict breathing and prevent the smooth circulation of blood and qi. Also, if the shoulders are not relaxed and the elbows are not dropped, it will make the guideline "arc your chest and round your back" impossible.

From a martial arts standpoint, drop the elbows is a protective strategy. If your shoulders are raised, your elbows will also be lifted. Also, when your elbows are too high, it will tense up your shoulders. When your shoulders are up, it is easier for your opponent to lift up your elbow, leaving the vital areas of your body exposed and vulnerable to an attack.

8.   Wrist and Hand: Extend the Fingers and Settle the Wrist (Zuo Wan Shen Zhi)

Extend the fingers and settle the wrist is a hand and wrist exercise. In settle the wrist, you are flexing your wrist by extending the base of your palm forward while leaving your fingertips suspended in place. Every time you settle your wrist and extend your fingers, the joints are being gently stretched and loosened. Energetically, the small motion of your wrist and hand helps bring your attention to your fingers, assisting your mind in leading the qi to your fingers.

From a martial arts standpoint, in a palm strike, the settling movement of your wrist increases the speed of your strike, which in turn increases the penetrating power of your strike. For example, if you were to throw a baseball at 50 mph, riding in the back of a pickup truck moving at 40 mph, neglecting air and all other resistance, the speed of the ball would be 90 mph (50 mph + 40 mph). This is the case with your arm thrusting forward (pickup speed) and settling your wrist (baseball speed) right before contacting your target.

9.   Legs: Distinguish Substantial and Insubstantial (Fen Qing Xu Shi)

Distinguish substantial and insubstantial is a guideline for the entire body. With regard to the leg movements, it is a guideline to achieve agility and smoothness in shifting weight from one leg to another. Substantial (*shi*) literally means "solid," implying firmness and stability, not rigidity. Insubstantial (*xu*) literally means "empty," implying the ability to change, not lifelessness.

Beginners often have the problem of falling into a stance, creating an abrupt change in movement and making balancing difficult. To prevent this from happening when stepping, do not step too wide or too far. Also, when your feet are too far apart, it will be very difficult for you to change stances. After touching down with your stepping foot, shift your weight forward gradually, paying attention to the weight transfer from the substantial leg to the insubstantial leg.

From a martial arts standpoint, as we have mentioned previously, "the root is at your feet; power is generated by your legs and directed by your waist, and then expressed through your fingers." Without the root, there is no balance. Without the proper transfer of weight, it is difficult to generate power from your legs.

10.   Entire Body: Upper and Lower Body Follow Each Other (Shang Xia Xiang Sui)

This guideline stresses the importance of integrating the entire body for good rooting, balance, and centering. When one part of your body moves, all other parts also move, providing a total body exercise.

The concept that your body moves as an integrated unit is often misunderstood to mean moving as one solid unit. A solid unit has to move unilaterally, while an integrated unit may move in any allowable direction. It is said in taijiquan that when there is an upward movement, then there is also a downward movement; when there is a forward movement, then there is also a backward movement; and when there is a left movement, then there is also a right movement. Energetically, your mind is aware of the movement of your entire body, balancing your body and qi in all directions, achieving total equilibrium of mind and body.

In terms of martial arts, when the movements of your legs don't coordinate with your arms, you make your legs ineffective for a defensive move or an attack. Similarly, when the movements of your arms don't coordinate with your legs, you make your arms ineffective for a defensive move or an attack. For example, your legs move within punching distance of your opponent, but your arms aren't set up with your legs to prepare for an attack. In this case, you not only lose the chance for an offensive move, but you also place yourself in striking distance for your opponent. Therefore, the movements must be accomplished simultaneously.

2.3: Guidelines for Breathing

Breathing is a process that we often take for granted. We never learned how to breathe; it simply came naturally when we were born. However, as we get older, due to a weakening and lack of exercise of the primary muscles associated with breathing, we begin to lose the full capacity of our lungs. Older individuals often find themselves breathing shallower and at a faster pace than they did when they were younger. This is primarily due to the loss of efficiency of the intercostal (rib) muscles and the diaphragm.

The mechanics of breathing have two phases: inhalation and exhalation. To inhale, the atmospheric pressure in the lungs must be lower than the atmospheric pressure of the environment. During inhalation, pressure in the lungs is reduced by lung expansion. This will increase the volume of the lungs, thereby reducing the pressure in the lungs, allowing the higher-pressured air from the outside to enter the lungs. To increase the volume of the lungs, the body contracts the diaphragm and intercostal muscles, to raise the ribs. Exhalation usually happens naturally by relaxing the contracted diaphragm and intercostal muscles. The relaxation of the intercostal muscles releases the elastic-like rib cage and pushes the air out of the lungs. As air is forced out of the lungs by the retraction of the rib cage, the differential pressure between the lung cavity and the abdominal cavity pulls the relaxed diaphragm upward. A relaxed diaphragm looks like an inverted bow pressing up on the bottom of the lungs.

In taijiquan practice, initially the breathing should be natural. That is, you are following the breathing pattern you are accustomed to. When your movements become smooth, then abdominal breathing is added to the postures. During abdominal breathing, abdominal muscles assist the intercostal muscles and the diaphragm in your breathing. During normal breathing, human lungs only exchange about 10 percent of the air in our lungs in each breathing cycle. That means we are diluting 10 percent of fresh air with 90 percent of residual air. As we get older, the air exchange rate becomes even less, due to the loss in the intercostal muscles and diaphragm efficiency. Abdominal breathing can help to make up the deficit and assist the intercostal muscles and the diaphragm in functioning more efficiently.

Abdominal breathing is also known as back to childhood breathing because, during childhood, children are able to breathe with the abdomen, making each breathing cycle more efficient. Pay attention to a young child during his or her sleep; you will notice that the child may still have the inherent ability to breath with his or her abdomen. There are two basic abdominal breathing practices. One is called normal abdominal breathing, and the other is called reverse abdominal breathing. In normal abdominal breathing, the abdomen is pushed out as you inhale and the abdomen is pulled in as you exhale. In reverse abdominal breathing, the abdomen is pulled in as you inhale and pushed out as you exhale. Generally speaking, normal abdominal breathing is more relaxed than reverse abdominal breathing. However, in reverse abdominal breathing, more air can be pushed out of the lungs, thereby allowing more air exchange in a breathing cycle.

Even though the term "reverse" is used to describe reverse abdominal breathing, it is still a natural way of breathing. Pay attention to how your abdomen reacts to your breathing while you attempt a physically demanding task, and you will notice your abdomen behaves in the fashion described for reverse breathing. For example, if you were to push a car stuck in a ditch, you would normally exhale while pushing and your abdomen would push out. This is a normal reaction for your body while doing a demanding task that requires a more efficient air exchange.

2.4: **Guidelines for Directing Your Mind (Yi) and Balancing Your Energy (Qi)**

Because the physical body and the mind act as an interrelated whole, any training of the physical body must include training of the mind. In taijiquan training, equal importance is placed on both parts of the whole. Physical exercise provides smooth paths for the mutual nourishment and mutual restraint of qi throughout the body. The conscious directing of your mind provides guidance for the flow of qi. During training, your mind is being trained to sense and lead the qi to specific areas of the body. This will heighten your body awareness, help regulate your qi, and help to increase your concentration. When conscious regulation becomes automatic, the flow of qi becomes smooth and natural—a state of regulating without regulating.

In Chinese, there are two different words for mind, *yi* and *xin*. These two terms refer to the inner workings of the mind. By directing your mind in sensing your qi, you are training your thought process. Chinese medicine classifies the expression of the spirit into seven emotions. They are joy, anger, worry, pensiveness, sadness, fear, and shock. When any of these emotions is excessive or lasts too long, the mind is unable to properly regulate it, destroying the energy in the organs, which then results in disease or illness.

In one of the earliest Chinese medical classics, *The Yellow Emperor's Internal Classics* (*Huangdi Neijing*), it states that excessive joy hurts the heart, excessive anger hurts the liver, being overly pensive hurts the spleen, excessive sorrow hurts the lungs, and excessive fear hurts the kidneys (see table on page 6: Some Correlations of the Five Elements). To balance, regulate, and prevent the buildup of excessive emotional tension, you may use your mind to direct your attention to specific areas of the body, or focus on an idea and/or applications, to prevent your thoughts from scattering.

1   Mind Focuses at Dan Tian (Yi Shou Dan Tian)

Dan tian literally means the "field of elixir." There are three places that are referred to as dan tian in the human body. They are the upper dan tian, located between the eyebrows; the middle dan tian, in the solar plexus area; and the lower dan tian, in the cavity within the abdomen. The lower dan tian is of primary concern in this discussion. When speaking of the lower dan tian as a specific point in the human body, it refers to the dan tian point located a little below the belly button. When speaking of lower dan tian as a "field of elixir," it refers to the area within the abdomen, around the center of gravity, which is capable of storing and generating qi.

The guideline *yi shou dan tian* points your mind to a central location in your body—the lower dan tian. The literal meaning of the word "shou" is to keep or to guard. It implies guarding your mind and qi to maintain their integrity and unity in your dan tian area, thus preventing the scattering of your thoughts and qi, in order to achieve harmony. The mind and qi are connected (*yi qi xiang li an*).

Yi shou dan tian is also a guideline for building qi in your dan tian. By paying attention to your dan tian, you will also be more aware of your abdominal movements. With practice, you will not only increase the efficiency of your breathing (see Guidelines for Breathing), but you will also be building qi in your dan tian. The expanding and contracting of your abdomen stimulates your kidneys (residence of your original essence), which helps produce qi to nourish your body.

2.   Use Your Mind to Lead the Qi (Yi Yi Ling Qi)

Qi can be led, not pushed. It is like a piece of rope that can be used to pull (lead), but not used to push an object. The mechanics of pulling with a rope requires that there be a pulling force ahead of the object bring pulled. *Yi yi ling qi* implies that your mind is the activator (force) that leads (pulls) the energy away from the excessive parts and leads it to the deficient parts, achieving a balance. To start this training, the mind focuses on specific points in the body, leading your sensation of qi toward that point. (In section 3.3, we will introduce the qi permeating technique that uses this guideline.) Another approach to this training is to place your mind on the martial applications of the taijiquan sequence. By being aware of the applications of the movements, your mind will be directing your qi toward your arms and legs, providing redistribution and balancing of qi. It's not crucial that you be aware of the martial applications, but the imagery elicited from the applications will also help direct the qi. For example, in a push posture, you can imagine you are pushing a car forward. The action of the push requires that you be firmly rooted (directing your mind downward) and you have placed your mind toward moving the car (directing your mind forward). This type of mental exercise leads the energy forward and back, dissipating excess tension and creating a balance.

CHAPTER THREE

Preparation Exercises and Qigong

3.1: **Introduction**

When doing any type of exercise, it is always advisable to do some simple warm-up exercises and stretching. It is not only important to get your physical body ready, but your mind must also be ready to exercise. This is especially true for taijiquan (tai chi chuan), since the intent of your mind leads the movements of your body. The following series of exercises will prepare you physically and mentally for your taijiquan training.

3.2: **Warm-up Exercises**

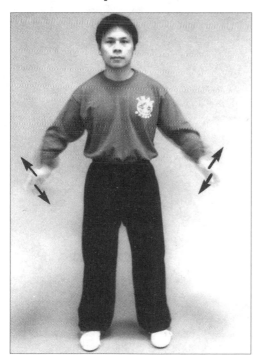

1. Shaking Arms: Stand with your feet shoulder width apart. Raise your forearms up slightly and gently shake your arms, loosening your wrist and elbow joints. Do this exercise for about ten seconds.

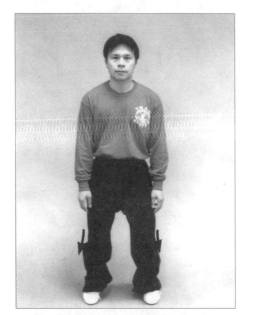
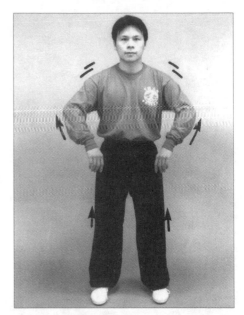

2. Shaking Body: Stand with your feet shoulder width apart and your arms placed naturally at your sides. Gently bounce your upper body up and down, bending and straightening your knees continuously. This warms up all your joints. Do this exercise for about ten seconds.

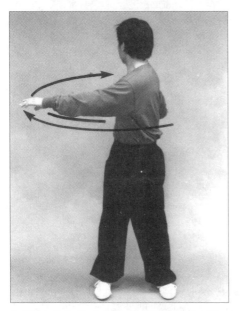
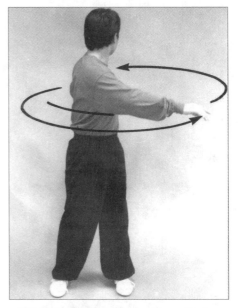

3. Swing Arms from Side to Side: Stand with your feet shoulder width apart. Swing both arms from side to side by turning your waist from left to right, then right to left. Don't allow your knees to move too much. This exercise is primarily for loosening your upper body. Moving your knees excessively is detrimental to your knees and reduces the effectiveness of this exercise. Do ten times on each side.

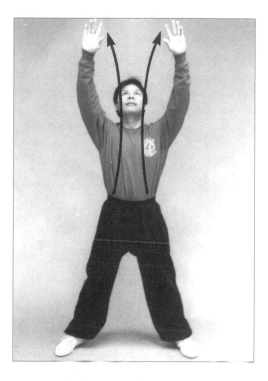

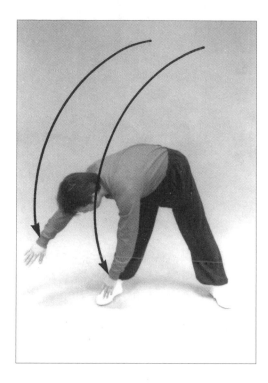

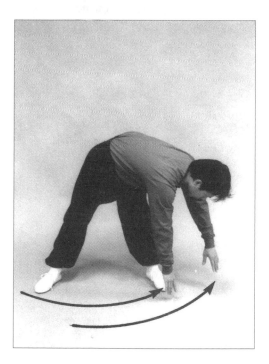

4. Upper Body Circle: Stand with your feet shoulder width apart. Stretch your hands over your head. Circle both arms to your right while bowing to your right and begin swinging your arms down. Continue swinging your arms down, then up to your left. Continue until your arms are back over your head. Repeat this exercise ten times; then change direction for another ten times.

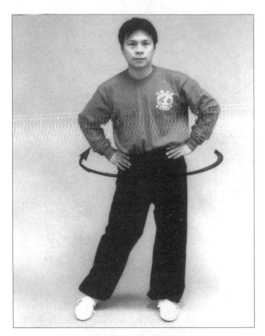

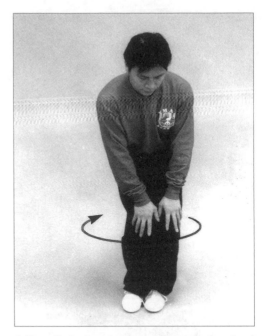

5. Waist Circle: Stand with your feet shoulder width apart. Place your hands on your waist and circle your waist clockwise for twenty rotations, and then counterclockwise twenty rotations. Keep your head in one place as you rotate your waist.

6. Knee Circle: Stand with your feet together. Bend your knees slightly and place your hands gently on top of your knees. Circle your knees clockwise for twenty rotations, and then counterclockwise for twenty rotations.

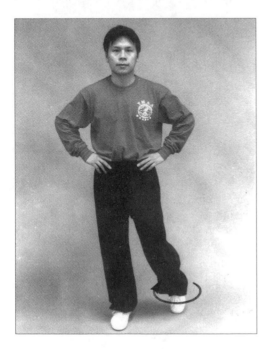

7. Ankle Circle: Place your hands on your waist and place the ball of your left foot slightly behind you. Then circle your left ankle twenty rotations clockwise and twenty rotations counterclockwise. Repeat this on the other leg. When doing this exercise, you should also keep your hip socket loose and relaxed.

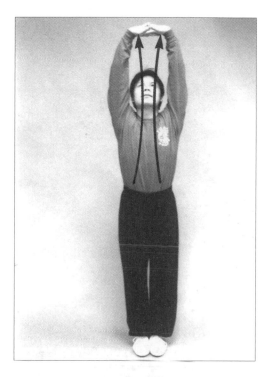

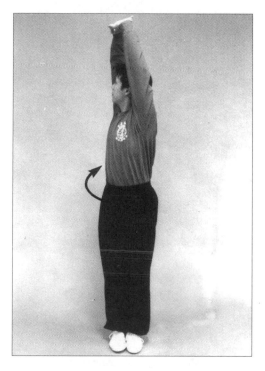

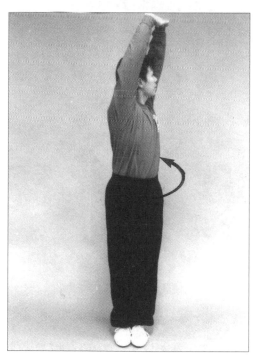

8. Spinal Stretch: Stand with your feet together, interlock your fingers, and push both palms up over your head. Slowly turn your body to your left, and then to your right; repeat.

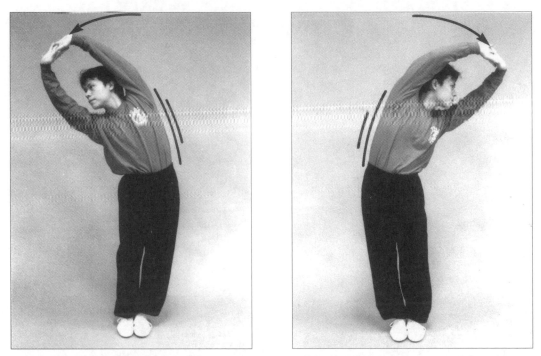

Face front and bend your body to your right. Bring your body back to the center, bend to your left, and repeat. Then repeat the entire sequence two more times. When doing this stretch, pay special attention to loosening your spine through stretching and rotating.

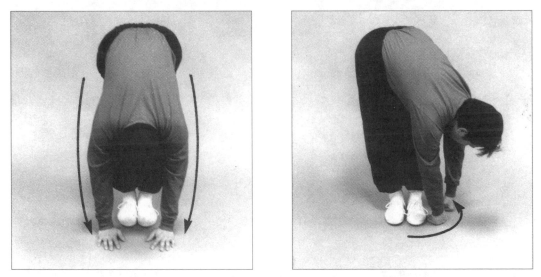

9. Touching the Floor: Stand with your feet together; slowly lower your hands down. Keep your legs straight as you lower your hands. Do this stretch slowly and only go as low as you can. Stay in this position for a few seconds; then turn your upper body to your left, and then to your right. To stand up, bend your knees slightly and stand up slowly. Repeat this sequence two more times.

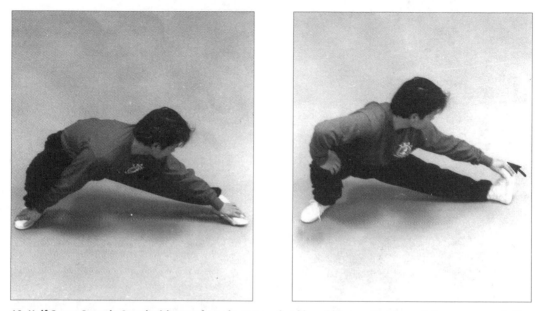

10. Half Squat Stretch: Stand with your feet about two shoulder widths apart and squat down on your right leg while keeping your left leg straight. Put your right hand on your right knee and left hand on your left foot. Hold this posture for twenty seconds, and then squat on the other leg for another twenty seconds. When doing this stretch, make sure your bent knee is pointing in the same direction as your foot. This will prevent your knee from being torqued. Squat down as low as you can without your heel coming off the floor. You may also do this stretch with your foot pointing up.

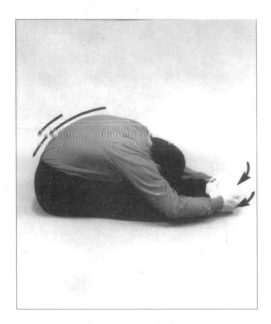

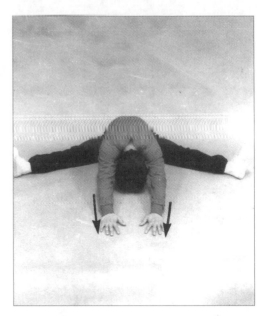

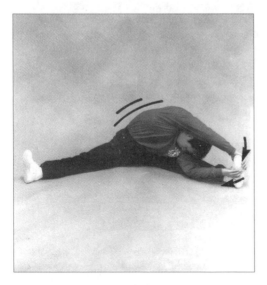

11. Floor Stretches: Sit on the floor with your legs extended forward. Bend over your legs and reach for your toes. Hold this posture for twenty seconds. Then open your legs to your sides. Again, bend over and reach forward with your hands. Hold this posture for twenty seconds. Turn to your left and reach your hands toward your left foot. Hold this posture for twenty seconds. Then turn to your right and reach your hands toward your right foot. Hold this posture for twenty seconds. As you do these two stretches, pay attention to your spine. Mentally loosen up one vertebra at a time.

3.3: **Qigong (Chi Kung)**

This qi permeating technique (*guan qi fa*) is the foundation of many qigong exercises. This simple exercise uses your mind to lead the qi through your body. It trains the mind to recognize and feel the body by paying attention to the paths and specific areas in your body. This exercise is done in a standing position. The palms follow your mind as you lead the qi down through your body. However, this exercise can also be done sitting or lying down. Use a slow, deep, relaxed breathing pattern.

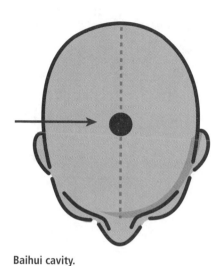

Baihui cavity.

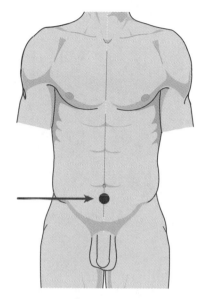

Dan tian cavity.

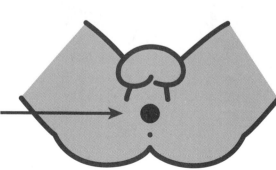

Huiyin cavity.

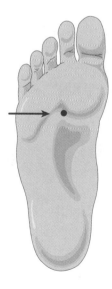

Yongquan cavity.

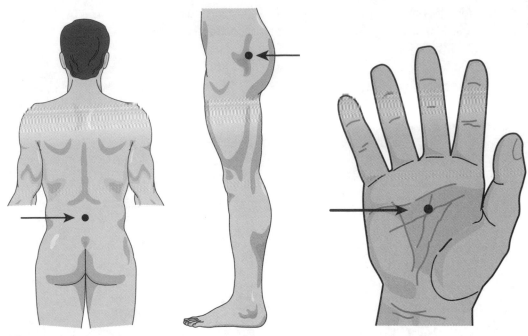

Mingmen cavity.   Huantiao cavity.   Laogong cavity.

Before learning this exercise, you should first visually locate the areas involved. The areas are baihui, on the top of your head; dan tian, slightly below your navel; *huiyin*, at the perineum—the area in front of your anus; *yongquan*, two-thirds of the way up the centerline of the foot, from your heel; *mingmen*, on your back around the fourteenth vertebra; *huantiao*, around the middle of your buttocks; and *laogong*, on your palm where your middle finger touches when holding a fist. Once you have located these areas, don't be overly concerned with pinpointing them exactly during the qigong exercise. What is important is to sense these areas with your mind.

Qi Permeating Technique (Guan Gi Fa)

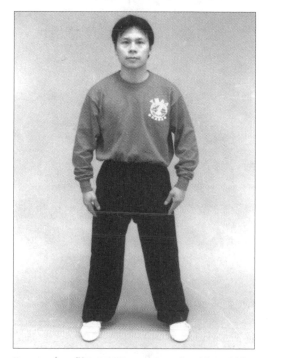 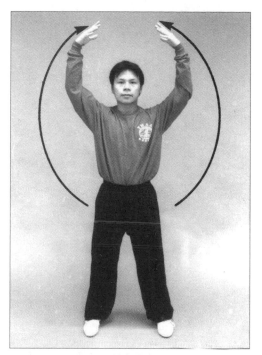

Preparation: Stand with your feet shoulder width apart with your palms naturally placed at your sides. Stand like this and breathe naturally until your mind is calm and your breathing is steady. Then raise both hands over your head with your laogong cavities pointing at your baihui cavity, and bend your knees slightly.

1. Front Path

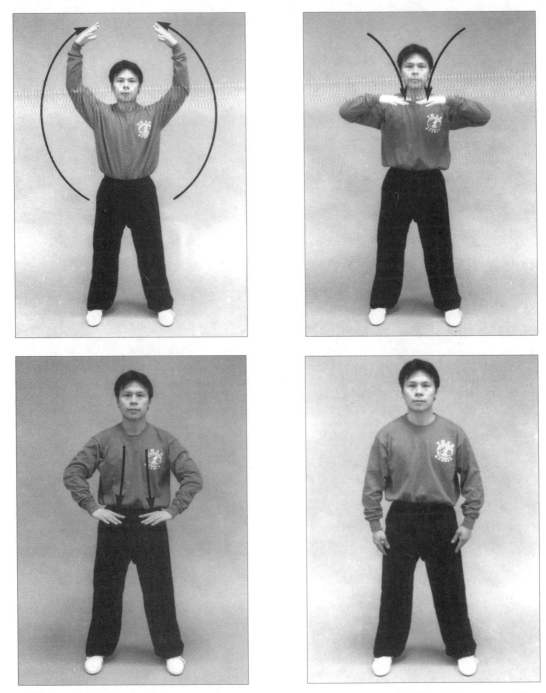

With your hands over your head, lower your palms in front of your body slowly until they are next to your sides.

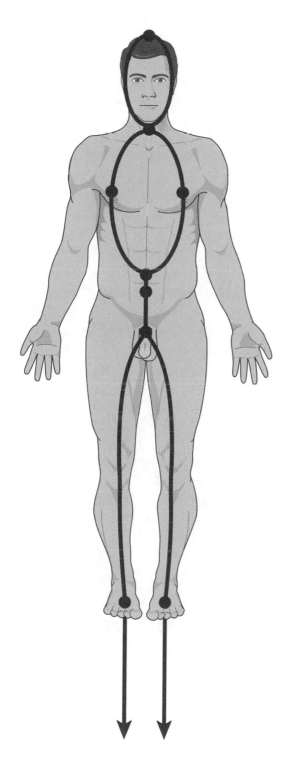

Front path.

As you use your mind to lead the qi down from your baihui, imagine that pure qi from the universe is filling your body. Divide into two paths, down past your ears and meeting at your throat. Again divide into two paths, down past your collar bones, to your nipples, and meeting at your belly button. Continue down to your dan tian and then to your huiyin. At this time, again separate into two paths down the inside of your legs. Imagine all your stress and tension are being led down through your yongquan until it is three feet into the ground. Feel and imagine that your body is filled with "pure qi" from the universe. Hold this position for a few seconds, and then repeat the exercise two more times. Start by lifting your hands up over your head.

2. Middle Path

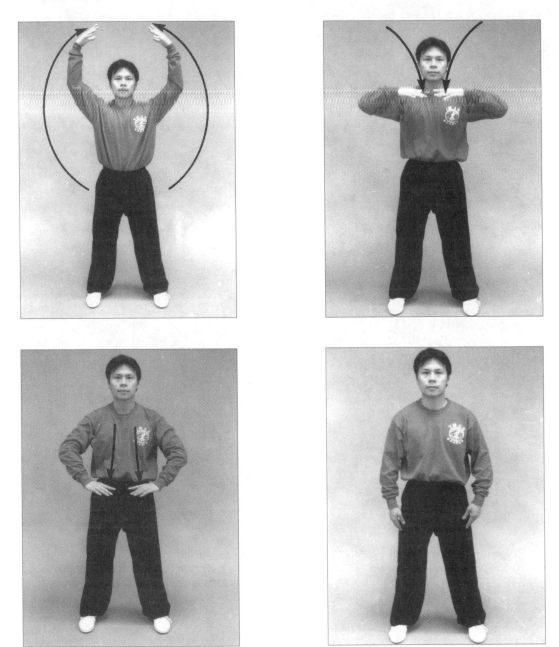

With your hands over your head, lower your palms in front of your body slowly until they are next to your sides, just as you did in the front path.

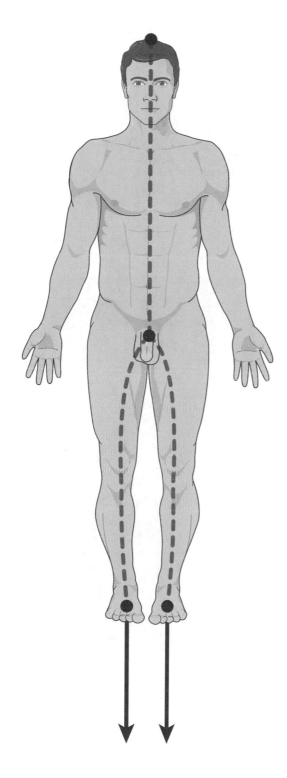

Middle path.

As you use your mind to lead the qi down from your baihui, imagine that pure qi from the universe is filling your body. Use your mind to lead the qi through your head, down the middle of your body, to your huiyin. At this time, imagine that all your stress and tension are being led down the bone marrow of your legs through your yongquan, and then three feet into the ground. Feel and imagine that your body is filled with pure qi from the universe. Hold this position for a few seconds, and then repeat the exercise two more times. Start by lifting your hands up over your head.

3. Back Path

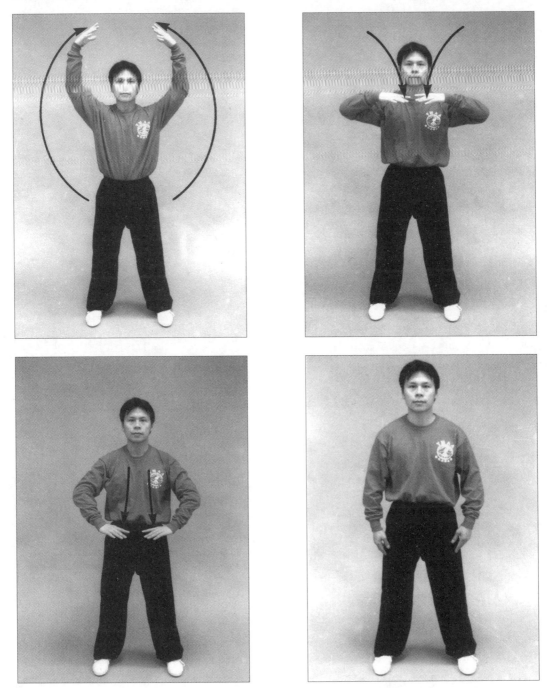

With your hands over your head, lower your palms in front of your body slowly, until they are next to your sides, just as you did in the front path.

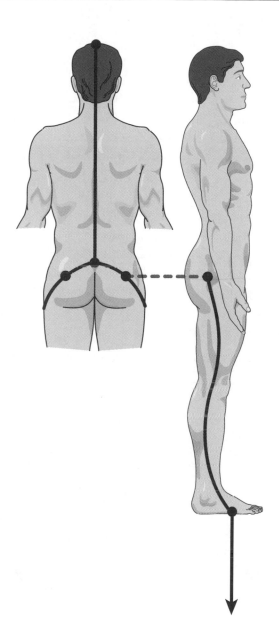

Back path.

As you use your mind to lead the qi down from your baihui, imagine that pure qi from the universe is filling your body. Use your mind to lead the qi down the back of your head to your neck, down along your spine to your mingmen. Then separate into two paths across your huantiao. At this time, imagine that all your stress and tension are being led down along the sides of your legs through your yongquan, three feet into the ground. Feel and imagine that your body is filled with pure qi from the universe. Hold this position for a few seconds, and then repeat the exercise two more times. Start by lifting your hands up over your head.

a. Each time you complete a cycle, visually loosen up every joint, muscle, and organ in your body (your head, neck, spine, shoulders, elbows, hands, hips, knees, feet, and internal organs). Then swallow your saliva, keep your body relaxed, and stand there for a few seconds before repeating the exercise.

b. If you practice only one of the three paths, do the path for nine cycles. If you do all three paths, then do each path for three cycles, a total of nine.

c. People who have high blood pressure should raise their hands over their head within a couple of seconds so there isn't too much energy brought up to the head and heart region.

d. People who have low blood pressure should raise their hands over their head slower than people who have high blood pressure.

e. The pace with which you lower your arms should feel comfortable and be slow enough to feel the points with your mind as you lower your hands.

f. After completing nine cycles, raise your heels off the floor and drop them down, stomping the floor. This will provide a gentle vibration throughout your body.

g. Breathe naturally; don't be concerned with abdominal breathing. You may keep your eyes closed, open, or half closed during this practice.

4. Finishing Touches

After completing the qigong exercises, your palms may feel the sensation of qi manifested as warmth or a tingling sensation. Place your palms next to each other, but not touching. Point your laogong cavities toward each other and see if you can feel the repulsion between your palms (another sensation of qi). If you do not feel it the first time, don't be overly concerned. It takes practice. Next, we will utilize the increase of qi to your palms to nourish parts of your body.

a. Face Massage: Rub your palms together about twenty times or until they are warm. Then place your palms on your face and slide both palms up over your head and down the back of your head to your neck. Repeat two more times. Then place your palms on your face again and slide your palms down your face to your neck. As you slide your palms down, press your middle fingers gently on the sides of your nose. Repeat two more times. This is a qigong approach for vitalizing the face, nourishing the lungs, and for helping to prevent the common cold.

b. Drumming the Head: Again, rub your palms together about twenty times or until they are warm. Then use your index fingers and thumbs to gently squeeze and rub your ears from top to bottom. The Chinese believe the ears contain the acupuncture points for the entire body. So stimulating the ears can provide a therapeutic effect on the whole body.

Next, place your palms over your ears and cross your index fingers over your middle fingers. Then slide your index fingers down your middle fingers and tap on the back of your head. This technique is known as "sounding the heavenly drum." You should feel and hear a drumming sound when your fingers tap on the back of your head. Do this a total of twenty-four times. This is a qigong approach for clearing the mind and vitalizing your spirit.

c. Eyes Exercise: Again, rub your palms together about twenty times or until they are warm. Then place your laogong cavities over your eyes. With your eyes closed, rotate your eyes clockwise, then counterclockwise, three to nine times in each direction. Remove your palms and look into the distance. This is an exercise for your eyes, which indirectly exercises your liver because of the relationship of your liver to your eyes.

d. Swallowing the Qi and Saliva: Once again, rub your palms together about twenty times or until they are warm. This time overlap your palms and place them over your mouth. With your mouth open, feel and swallow the warm qi and your saliva into your stomach. This is a qigong approach to nourish the stomach and intestines.

After completing these qi permeating techniques, walk around for a few minutes. Continue with your taijiquan practice, noticing your heightened sensation of qi.

3.4: **Stationary, Moving Stances, and Hand Forms**

Proper alignment of your legs and the transfer of weight from one leg to another are very important in taijiquan practice. Like any other exercise, improper alignment can cause ligament damage. Improper alignment also prevents you from attaining the physical centering required for proper qi balancing in your body.

Stationary Stances

1. Horse Stance (Ma Bu)

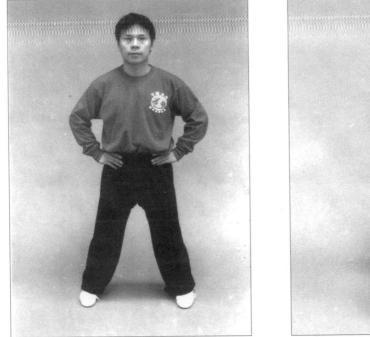 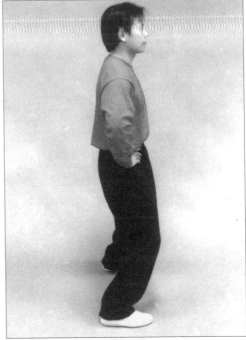

This stance resembles a person riding on a horse, thus it is called horse stance. When practicing this stance, stand with your feet parallel and about shoulder width apart. Bend both knees slightly. Keep your back straight and tuck your sacrum in slightly. Your weight should be evenly distributed on both feet. When standing in *ma bu,* keep your knees pointing in the same direction as your feet. Do not allow your knees to rotate out and create undue stress on them. If you feel your knees are in torsion, you may turn your foot out slightly instead of keeping them parallel; or you may keep your feet parallel, but squeeze your knees in slightly until they are in alignment with your feet.

2. Bow Stance (Gong Bu)

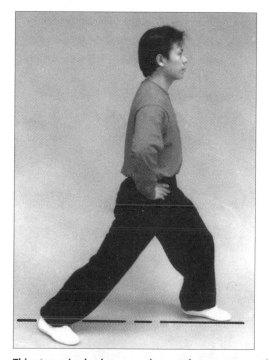 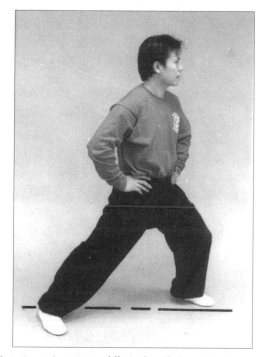

This stance is also known as bow and arrow stance. The front leg is bent, resembling a bow being pulled, and the back leg is straight, resembling an arrow on the bow. When practicing a left bow stance, stand with your left foot in front of your right foot, about one and a half times your shoulder width apart. Both feet point to your front right corner. Your back foot turns in about 45 degrees, and the front foot turns in slightly. Your left knee is bent, but not extending over your right foot, and your right leg extends straight, without locking your knee. If you draw a line from front to back, your right foot would be on the right side of the line, and your left heel on the left side of the line. Your weight should be about 70 percent on the bent leg and 30 percent on the straight leg. The left bow stance is a mirror image of the right.

The picture shows your body facing forward. The full name for this stance is straight bow stance (*zheng gong bu*). This stance is generally associated with postures that require the arm to be extended opposite to the front leg. If your body is facing forward at an angle, the full name would be slant bow stance (*xie gong bu*). Slant bow stance is generally associated with postures that require the arm to be extended on the same side as the front foot.

3. Empty Stance (Xu Bu)

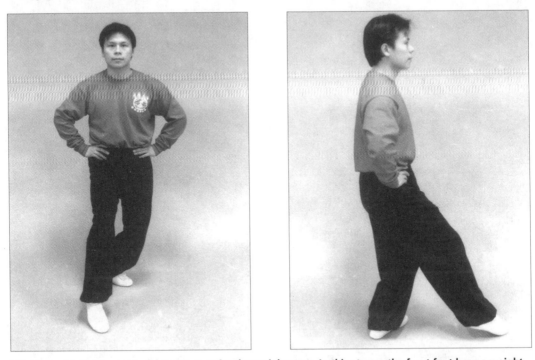

This stance is also known as false stance or insubstantial stance. In this stance, the front foot has no weight on it, therefore giving the stance the name empty, false, or insubstantial. When practicing empty stance on the right side, turn your left foot about 45 degrees out and put all your weight on your left leg. Then place your right foot in front of your left about a shoulder width apart, touching down on the ball of your foot. The ball of your right foot should be directly in front of your left heel, with your right heel turned out slightly. When your right heel turns out, your right knee will automatically turn in slightly. This is empty stance on the right side.

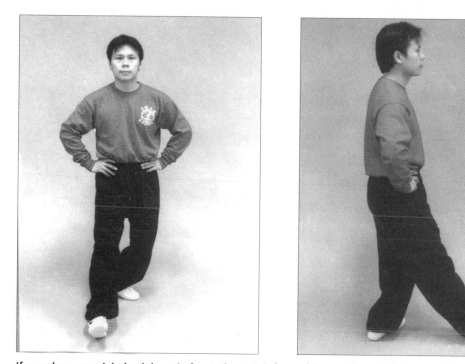

If you place your right heel down in front of your left foot, with your foot pointing up, it would be called empty stance on your heel. In this empty stance, the front leg should be completely relaxed. Empty stance on the left side is simply the mirror image of the right side.

4. Half Squat Stance (Pu Bu)

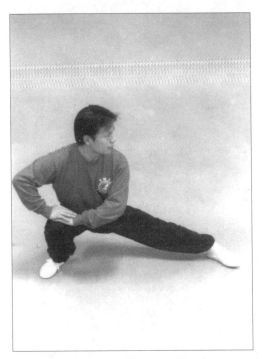 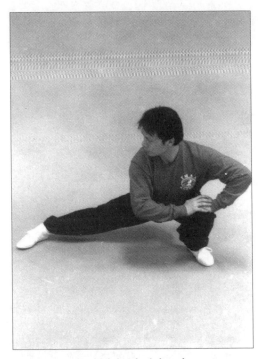

This stance requires that you squat down on one leg, close to the ground, which is why it has the name *pu bu,* meaning down to the ground stance. It is important for beginners to gradually go lower in stances. Do not attempt low stances right away. When practicing this stance on the right side, stand with your feet about two shoulder widths apart with the feet pointing out slightly. Then turn your upper body slightly to your left and squat down on your right leg while keeping your left leg straight. To change to the left side, shift your weight to your left leg and squat down on it while you straighten your right leg. To prevent your knee from being torqued while practicing this stance, it is important that the knee of your bent leg be pointing in the same direction as your foot.

5. Resting Stance (Xie Bu)

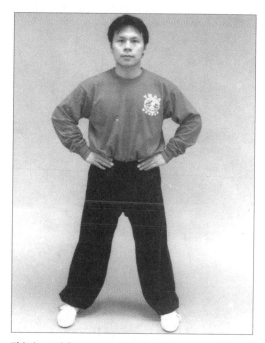

This is a tricky stance. This stance is not used in the 24 Posture Taijiquan sequence, but it is used in the 48 Posture Taijiquan sequence. When practicing this stance with your left foot forward, first stand with your feet shoulder width apart.

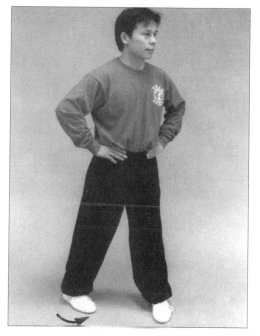

Turn your right foot in, about 45 degrees.

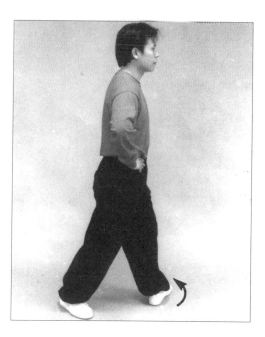

Then turn your left foot to your left.

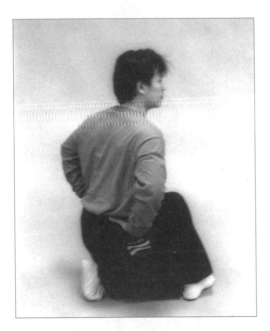

Bend your left knee over your left foot as you sink your body down, and bring your right knee behind your left calf.

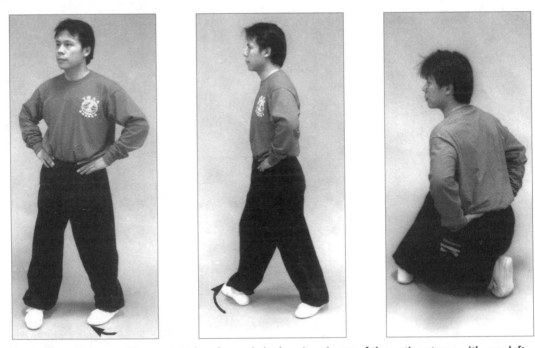

To practice this stance with your right foot forward, do the mirror image of the resting stance with your left foot forward.

6. Sit Back Stance (Zuo Bu)

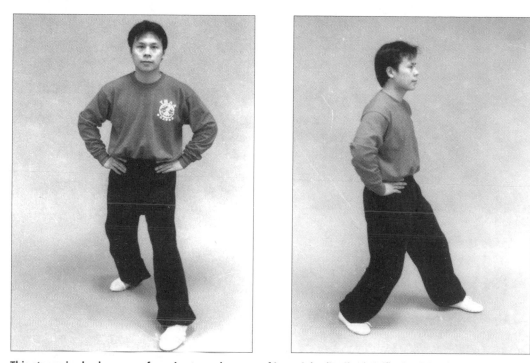

This stance is also known as four six stance because of its weight distribution. The back leg has 60 percent of the weight and the front leg has 40 percent of the weight. It is a transitional stance for many other stances due to its flexibility for changing from one stance to another. When practicing a sit back stance with your left foot in front of your right foot, first stand a little wider than shoulder width apart, with both feet pointing to your front right corner. Put about 60 percent of your weight on your back leg and tuck your sacrum in slightly. This stance resembles a person sitting on a chair. Make sure your right knee is pointing in the same direction as your right foot. The right side of this stance is the mirror image of this one.

7. Single Leg Stance (Du Li Bu)

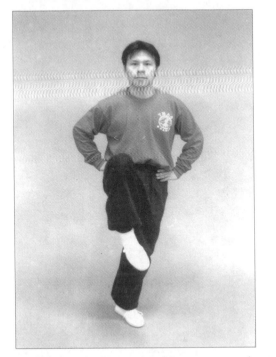 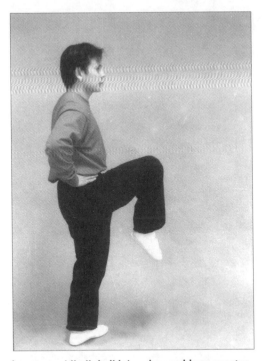

This stance is also known as golden rooster stands on one leg stance (*jin ji du li bu*) and resembles a rooster standing on a perch with one leg propped up. This stance is important for balance training. It trains your awareness of your center of gravity and aligns your body. Imagine you are a tree deeply rooted into the ground. When practicing a left single leg stance, start by standing with your feet together, and then turn your left foot out about 45 degrees. Next, lift your right knee up as high as you can. Keep your right foot naturally dropped. Do not flex your foot.

Moving Stances

1. Forward Movements: Bow Stance to Bow Stance

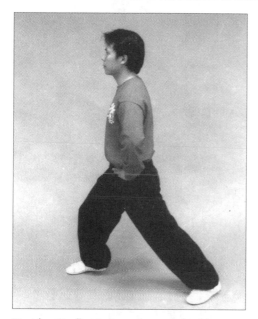

Start by standing in bow stance, right side.

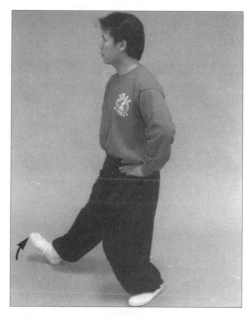

Shift your weight back to your left leg.

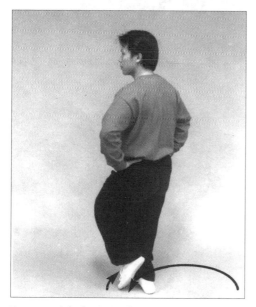

Turn your right foot out about 45 degrees and bring your left foot next to your right foot.

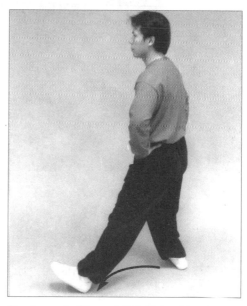

Step forward with your left foot, touching down on your heel.

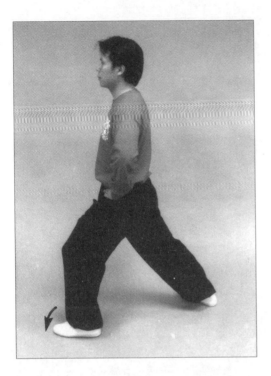

Shift your weight forward into bow stance left side. When stepping forward, make sure you don't cross your legs by stepping too far to your right.

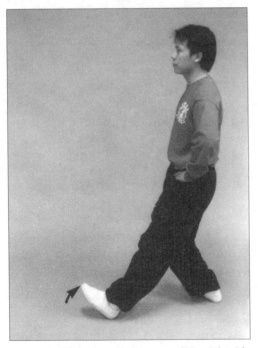

Repeat by doing the mirror image of the right side.

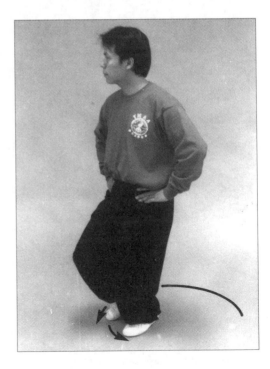

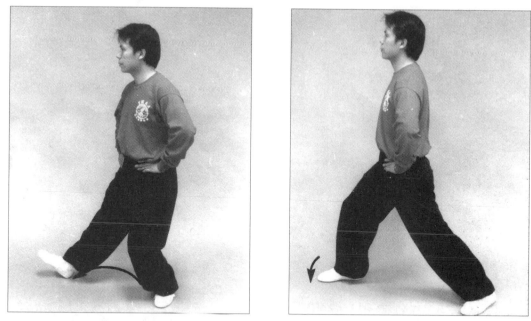

Repeat by doing the mirror image of the right side (continued).

2. Backward Movements: Sit Back Stance to Sit Back Stance

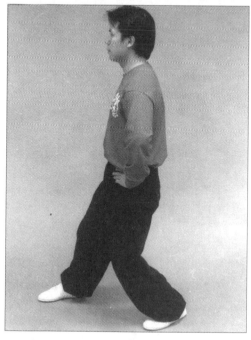

Start by standing in sit back stance with your right foot forward.

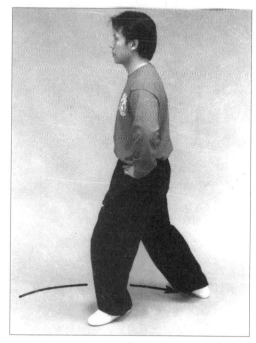

Step back with your right foot touching down with the ball of your right foot first.

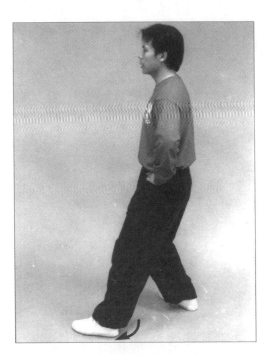

Shift your weight back to your right leg. Then turn your left heel out. When stepping backward, make sure you don't cross your legs by stepping too far to your left.

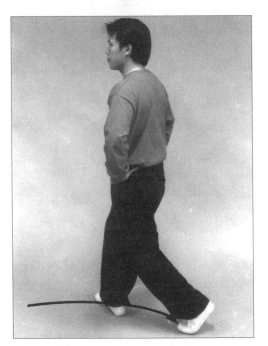

Repeat by doing the mirror image of the right side.

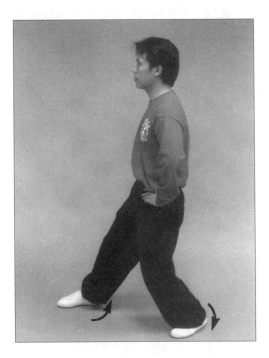

3. Sideward Movements: Horse Stance to Horse Stance

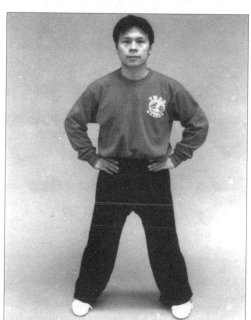

Start by standing in horse stance.

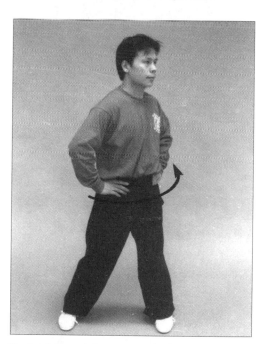

To step to your left, turn your body to your left while shifting your weight to your left leg.

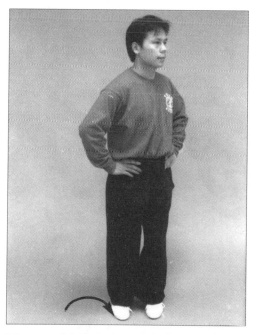

Bring your right foot about six inches away from your left foot.

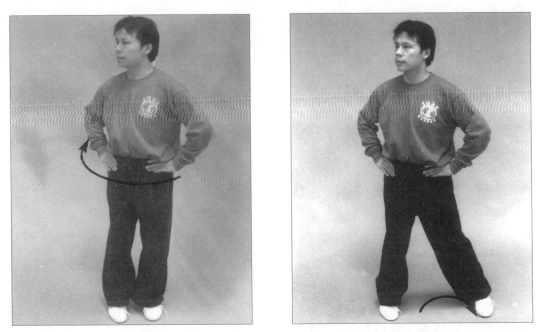

Turn your body to your right and step to your left with your left foot. Turn your body back to face forward in horse stance; then repeat the exercise from the beginning.

4. Changing Directions: Bow Stance to Bow Stance

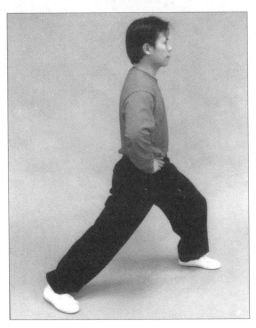

Start by standing in a left bow stance.

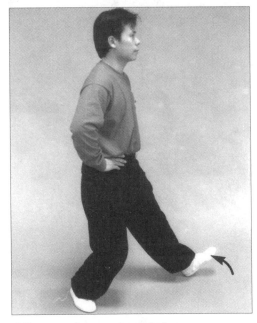

Shift your weight on your right leg.

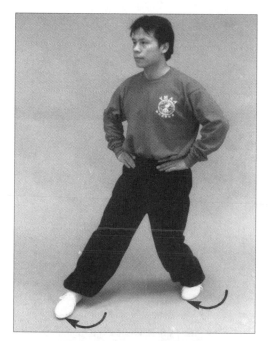

Turn your left foot in and right foot out as you shift your weight back to your left leg.

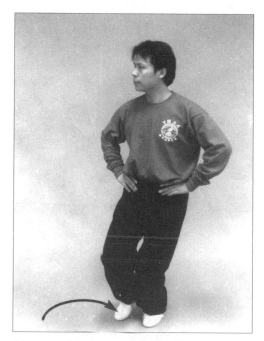

Bring your right foot next to your left.

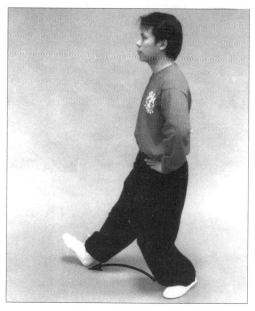

Step forward, slightly to your right with your right foot, touching down on your heel.

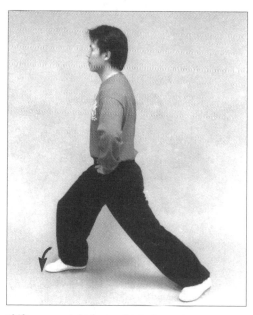

Shift your weight forward into bow stance.

Hand Forms

1. Palm (Zhang)

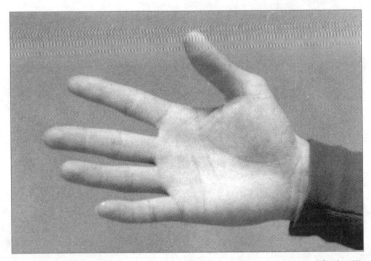

The natural position of your palm is with your fingers slightly bent in. In the Simplified Taijiquan and the 48 Posture Taijiquan, the palm is used by extending your fingers slightly, with your fingers naturally spaced apart. If you were holding a basketball, the entire palm would be in contact with the surface of the ball. That is, the palm should be rounded and appear full of energy.

2. Fist (Quan)

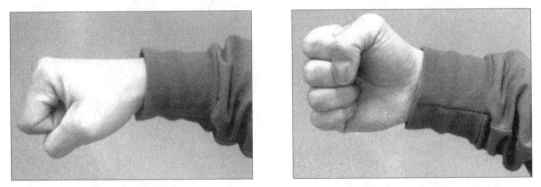

From an open palm, fold your fingers in, one section at a time, and place your thumb on top of the second section of your index and middle fingers. For all straight punches, keep your wrist even with your forearm and knuckles. When holding a fist, you want a firm grip, but not a tight grip. Imagine you have a fragile piece of pencil lead in your palm. If you hold your fist too tight, you will break the lead. If you hold it too loose, the lead will fall out of your hand.

3. Hook (Gou)

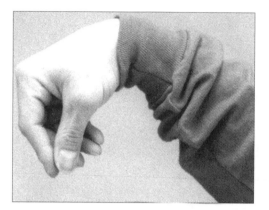

From an open palm facing down, squeeze the base of your thumb in slightly. Then hook your fingers down one at a time, starting with your pinky, until all your fingers are together, pointing down. By moving your fingers individually, you are exercising the joints in your hand.

CHAPTER FOUR

24 Posture Taijiquan with Applications

4.1: **Introduction**

Simplified Taijiquan (Tai Chi Chuan) was compiled by the Chinese Sports Commission in 1956 with the goal of standardizing and popularizing taijiquan. It consists of twenty different postures from the Yang Style Long Sequence. Three of the postures are done on both left and right sides, and one of the postures repeats itself, making a total of twenty-four postures. This is why it is also commonly referred to as 24 Posture Taijiquan. Because this sequence is based on Yang Style Taijiquan, the training guidelines and principles of Simplified Taijiquan follow the characteristic "flavor" of the Yang Style. The entire Simplified Taijiquan sequence should be performed at an even pace, with no abrupt changes in the transition, and should follow the guidelines and principles outlined in chapter two.

It is never an easy task to learn from a book. When following the instructions in this book, it is important to remember they are presented with as much relevant information as possible. For beginners, there may be too many details to assimilate at one time. In classroom instruction, the instructor often tells students to pay attention to only one or two aspects of the sequence at a time. As students get better at the primary aspects of the sequence, the teacher will then introduce more aspects of the movements. As you learn from this book, it is recommended that you do the same—focus on one aspect at a time. You might want to read the entire book before attempting to learn the postures. Many of the key points are explained after the movement descriptions. Some of the unclear parts of the photographs are further clarified by mirror images of the postures. When you begin to learn the postures, don't be overly concerned with coordinating your breathing with the movements. Once your movements are smooth, start to pay attention to your breathing. Then reread the principles described in chapter two and try to incorporate them into the entire sequence.

4.2: **24 Posture Taijiquan with Key Points and Applications**

24 Posture Taijiquan (Simplified Taijiquan) Posture Names

1. Commencing (*Qi Shi*)
2. The Wild Horse Parts Its Mane (*Ye Mu Fen Zong*)
3. White Crane Spreads Its Wings (*Bai He Liang Chi*)
4. Brush Knee and Step Forward (*Lou Xi Ao Bu*)
5. Playing the Lute (*Shou Hui Pipa*)
6. Reverse Reeling Forearm (*Dao Juan Gong*)
7. Left Grasp Sparrow's Tail (*Zuo Lan Que Wei*)
8. Right Grasp Sparrow's Tail (*You Lan Que Wei*)
9. Single Whip (*Dan Bian*)
10. Wave Hands Like Clouds (*Yun Shou*)
11. Single Whip (*Dan Bian*)
12. High Pat on Horse (*Gao Tan Ma*)
13. Right Heel Kick (*You Deng Jiao*)
14. Strike to Ears with Both Fists (*Shuang Feng Guan Er*)
15. Turn Body and Left Heel Kick (*Zhuan Shen Zuo Deng Jiao*)
16. Left Lower Body and Stand on One Leg (*Zuo Xia Shi Du Li*)
17. Right Lower Body and Stand on One Leg (*You Xia Shi Du Li*)
18. Shuttle Back and Forth (*Chuan Suo*)
19. Needle at Sea Bottom (*Haidi Zhen*)
20. Fan through Back (*Shan Tong Bei*)
21. Turn Body, Deflect, Parry, and Punch (*Zhuan Shen Ban Lan Chui*)
22. Appears Closed (*Ru Feng Si Bi*)
23. Cross Hands (*Shi Zi Shou*)
24. Closing (*Shou Shi*)

24 Posture Taijiquan movement chart

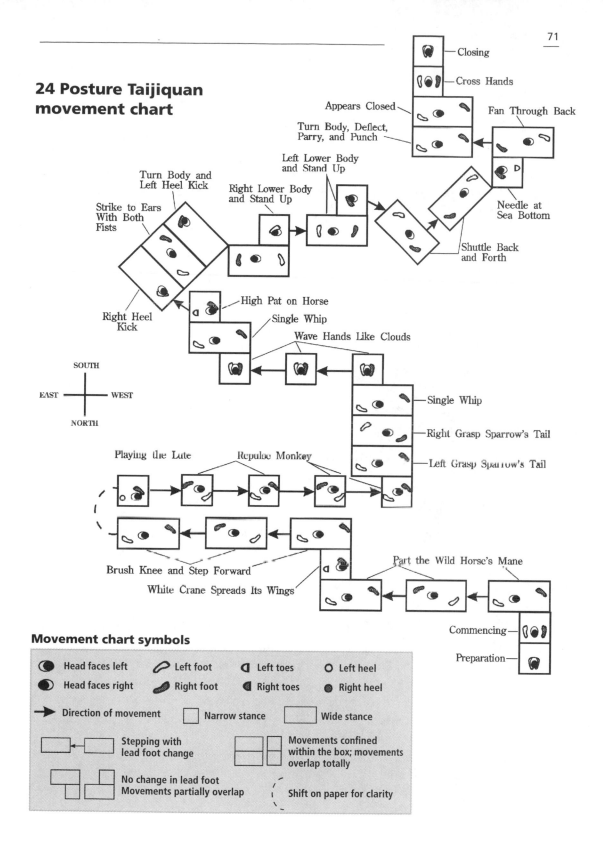

Closing

Cross Hands

Appears Closed

Fan Through Back

Turn Body, Deflect, Parry, and Punch

Left Lower Body and Stand Up

Right Lower Body and Stand Up

Needle at Sea Bottom

Turn Body and Left Heel Kick

Strike to Ears With Both Fists

Shuttle Back and Forth

Right Heel Kick

High Pat on Horse

Single Whip

Wave Hands Like Clouds

SOUTH

EAST — WEST

NORTH

Single Whip

Right Grasp Sparrow's Tail

Left Grasp Sparrow's Tail

Playing the Lute

Repulse Monkey

Brush Knee and Step Forward

White Crane Spreads Its Wings

Part the Wild Horse's Mane

Commencing

Preparation

Movement chart symbols

- ◖ Head faces left
- ◗ Head faces right
- ➤ Direction of movement

- Left foot
- Right foot

- ◐ Left toes
- ◑ Right toes
- ▢ Narrow stance

- ○ Left heel
- ● Right heel
- ▢ Wide stance

Stepping with lead foot change

No change in lead foot Movements partially overlap

Movements confined within the box; movements overlap totally

Shift on paper for clarity

Preparation

In this book, we will face south as the reference point for the starting position. We suggest that you refer to the 24 Posture Taijiquan movement chart that shows footprints and directional arrows, along with the movement chart symbols. The starting and ending positions are relatively in the same location. For the sake of clarity, we have drawn the movements above each other instead of overlapping. This is the reason for the large area covered with movements, when in fact the entire sequence is done overlapping in a rectangular space.

Movements

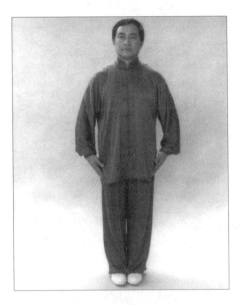

Stand with feet together and hands to your sides. (Face south. Inhale and exhale naturally a few times.)

Key Points

Training the mind is of the highest importance in taijiquan. The preparation posture is to prepare the mind for the physical movements. Before starting the movements, the mind should be calm and steady. Stand naturally upright. Bring your thoughts inward instead of outward. Eyes look evenly forward. Relax your entire body. Imagine there is a waterfall gently pouring over your head. As the water passes through your body, tension is released in your head, neck, shoulders, chest, spine, elbows, hands, hips, knees, ankles, feet, and toes—and then into the ground. Repeat this process until you feel completely relaxed and calm.

Before starting the postures, touch your tongue to the roof of your mouth. As saliva is being generated, swallow it and use your mind to follow the saliva down your throat to your stomach. Then bring your attention to your dan tian—your body's center of gravity.

SECTION I

Posture 1: Commencing (Qi Shi)

Movements

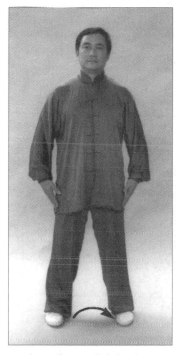 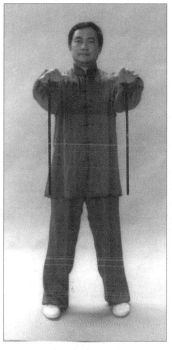 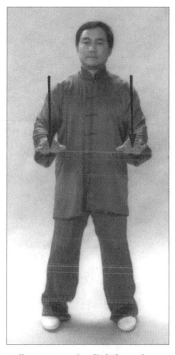

Bend your knees slightly. Then step to your left with your left leg, shoulder width apart. (Begin to inhale.)

Rotate your palms as you raise your arms up slowly to shoulder level, palms facing down.

Pull your arms in slightly and lower them to abdomen level as you bend your knees slightly. (Exhale.)

Key Points

When moving your arms up and down, do not let your elbows extend too far to the sides, nor should the elbows be locked. When lowering your arms, the elbows should be lowered slightly before the hands. This will create a wavelike movement in your arms, making the movements rounded and smooth. The bending of your knees and lowering of your hands should be done simultaneously.

Commencing posture refers to the beginning of the sequence. It can be thought of as the starting move. It can also be a martial technique. As the arms move up, they can intercept an opponent's punch. As the arms begin to move down, the palms can strike forward to counterattack the opponent. When training this posture as a martial technique, you must train the movements repeatedly to achieve the effectiveness of the technique. This is true for all martial techniques. When you train a single posture repeatedly, it is called single posture training (*dan lian*).

When you lower your hands, imagine you are pushing an object down with your palms. As your body lowers, imagine you are immersing your body into the deepest part of the ocean. Do not bend your knees excessively or extend over your toes. Go as low as your legs can handle without leaning forward with your body. Your weight should be evenly distributed between your legs.

Application

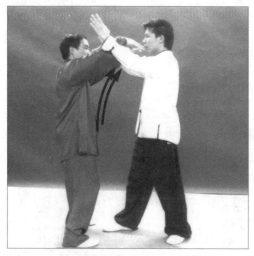

White attempts to grab Gray's neck with both hands. Gray raises both arms and intercepts White's arms with his forearms.

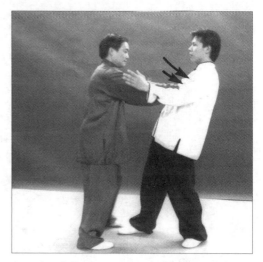

Gray then follows up with a double palm strike to White's chest.

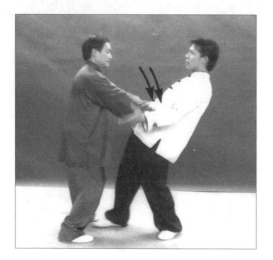

As an alternative, Gray could seal White's arms down by pressing his palms down on White's elbows and throwing him off balance.

Posture 2: The Wild Horse Parts Its Mane (Ye Ma Fen Zong)

Movements

The Wild Horse Parts Its Mane, left side

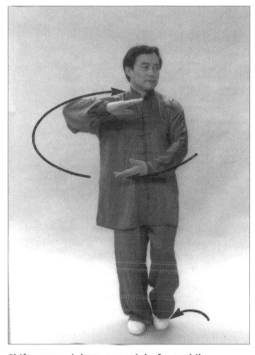 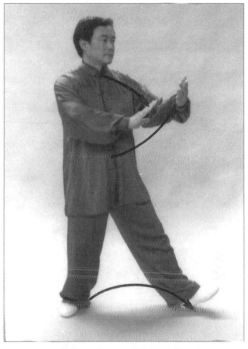

Shift your weight to your right foot while touching your left foot next to your right. Turn your body slightly to your right, and then back again while circling both palms counterclockwise and rotating them to face each other. The palms resemble the embrace of a ball in front of your chest. Eyes look in the same direction as your right hand. (Inhale.)

Step to your left with your left foot, touching down with your heel first. Begin turning your body to your left while pulling your right hand down and extending your left hand forward. (Step east. Begin to exhale.)

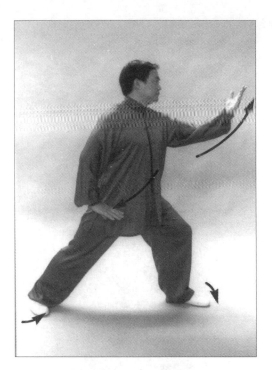

Shift your weight forward into a left bow stance while extending your left palm forward until it is at eye level and lowering your right palm until it is next to your hip. (Face east.)

The Wild Horse Parts Its Mane, right side

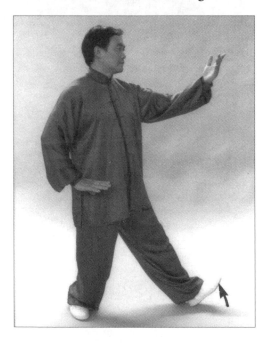

Shift your weight back to your right foot. Lift up the ball of your left foot. (Begin to inhale.)

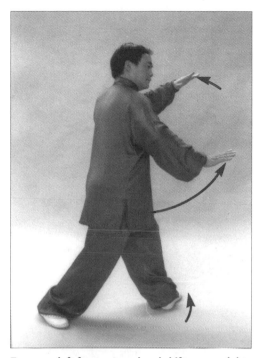

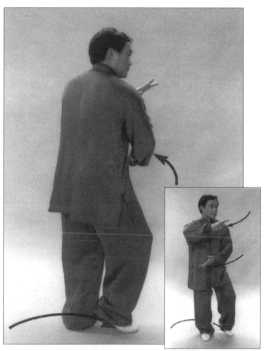

Turn your left foot outward and shift your weight on it while you begin to turn your body to your left. Rotate your left palm until it is facing down and let your right hand circle forward with the rotation of your body. Eyes gaze in the direction of your left hand.

Bring your right foot forward next to your left while bringing your left palm next to your chest, palm down, and bringing your right palm next to your abdomen, palm up. (See mirror image.)

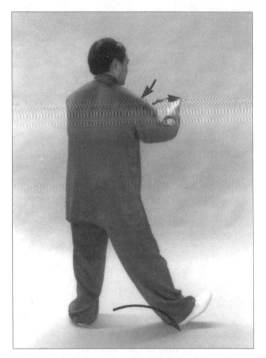

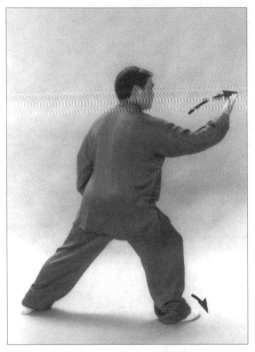

Step forward with your right foot, touching down with your heel first. Begin turning your body to your right while pulling your left hand down and extending your right hand forward. (Begin to exhale.)

Shift your weight forward into a right bow stance while extending your right palm forward until it is at eye level and lowering your left palm until it is next to your hip. (Face east.)

The Wild Horse Parts Its Mane, left side

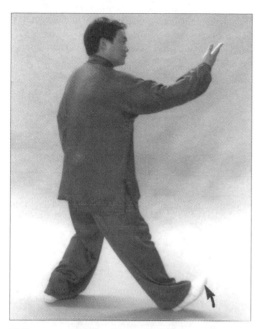

Shift your weight back to your left foot. Lift up the ball of your right foot. (Begin to inhale.)

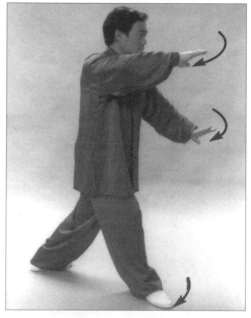

Turn your right foot out and shift your weight on it while you begin to turn your body to your right. Rotate your right palm until it is facing down, and let your left hand circle forward with the rotation of your body. Eyes look in the direction of your right hand.

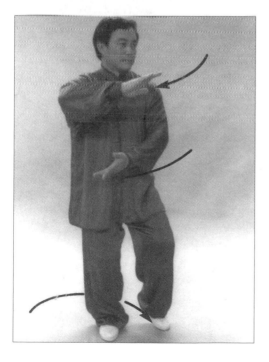

Bring your left foot forward next to your right while bringing your right palm next to your chest, palm down, and bringing your left palm next to your abdomen, palm up.

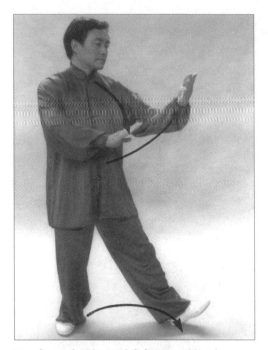

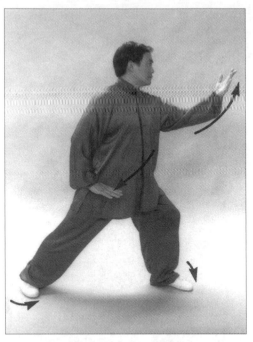

Step forward with your left foot, touching down with your heel first. Begin turning your body to your left while pulling your right hand down and extending your left hand forward. (Begin to exhale.)

Shift your weight forward into a left bow stance while extending your left palm forward until it is at eye level and lowering your right palm until it is next to your hip. (Face east.)

Key Points

Do not allow your upper body to lean forward or backward. Your chest should be naturally open and relaxed. When extending the arms apart, maintain a circular extension. The waist should lead the rotation of the upper body. Make sure when you step into the bow stance, your feet are not in a straight line. The front foot and the back foot should be on each side of the centerline. When stepping into the bow stance, make sure the heel touches down first, and then gradually shift your weight to the front leg. Do not fall into the stance. The back leg naturally extends until it is straight, but not locked. The angle formed with the front foot and back foot should not exceed 90 degrees. When necessary, adjust your back foot to match.

The wild horse parts its mane has the implication of separating the horse's mane. The palms pass each other as they move in separate directions. The horse's mane is separated by the wind as it heads into the wind. It is as though a wild horse were galloping freely in the prairie, releasing all cooped-up tension and stress. As you do this posture, imagine you are throwing a Frisbee. As you extend your arms, pay attention to the muscles in your body being stretched loose and the energy allowed to flow freely.

Applications

First application

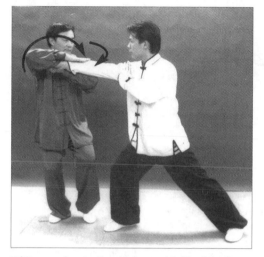

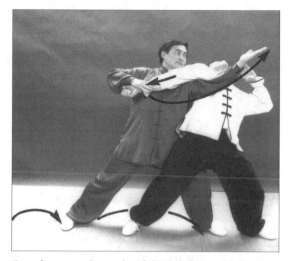

White punches to Gray's chest with his right fist. Gray intercepts with his left forearm and brings his right palm over White's forearm.

Gray then steps forward with his left foot behind White. At the same time, Gray grabs hold of White's right wrist with his right hand and extends his left arm up from under White's right arm. Notice that White's elbow is locked tightly on Gray's chest and White's shoulder is elevated by Gray's shoulder.

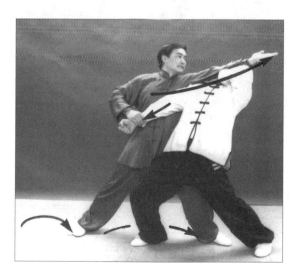

As an alternative, Gray could extend his left arm up from above White's right arm toward White's neck. Notice that White's right elbow is locked tightly on Gray's chest and Gray's arm is pressing down on White's neck.

Second application

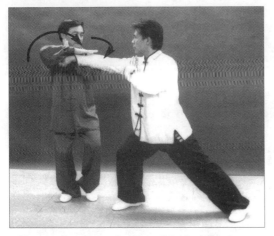

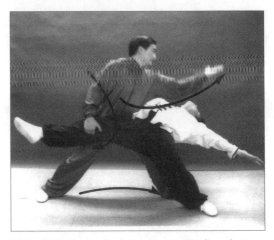

White punches to Gray's chest with his right arm. Gray intercepts with his left forearm and brings his right palm over White's forearm, attempting to grab hold of White's wrist.

White pulls his arm back to prevent Gray's grab. Gray then steps behind White and extends his left arm toward White's neck while grabbing the inside of White's knee and pulling it up. This pulls White off balance and makes him fall.

Third application

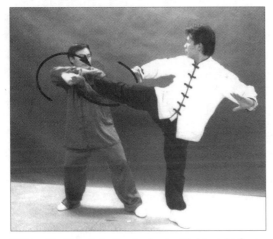

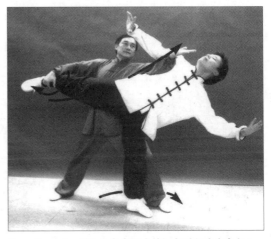

White side kicks into Gray's chest with his right foot. Gray scoops White's leg up with his left forearm and brings his right palm over White's foot.

Gray then steps his left foot behind White's left leg while hooking onto White's shin with his right hand and extends his left palm toward White's neck. Notice that Gray's left knee locks White's left leg in place, preventing White from escaping.

Posture 3: White Crane Spreads Its Wings (Bai He Liang Chi)

Movements

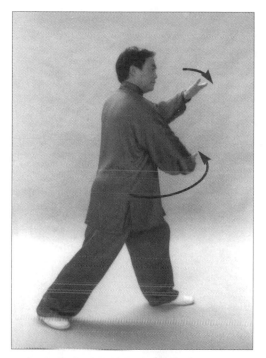 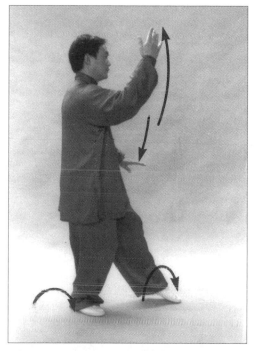

Turn your body slightly to your left while extending your right palm forward and rotating both palms until they face each other. Right palm faces up; left palm faces down. (Inhale.)

Bring your right foot a half step forward. Shift all your weight onto your right foot. At the same time, bring your right palm up past your left elbow and lift your left foot up slightly. Complete the movement by lowering your left palm down to waist level, palm down. Raise your right palm up to head level, palm facing inward, and touch down with your left foot into empty stance. (Exhale.)

Key Points

White crane spreads its wings is describing the beauty of the crane's wings. When you wear the traditional Chinese outfit to do this posture, it appears as though you are a crane spreading its wings. It is very pleasing to the eyes. At the completion of this posture, do not allow your chest to be overly extended. Both of your arms should be rounded. The shifting of your weight backward, the lowering of your left palm, and the raising of your right palm should all be completed simultaneously. As you do this posture, imagine you are a crane standing against the wind with your wings extended, radiating with confidence and strength.

Applications

First application

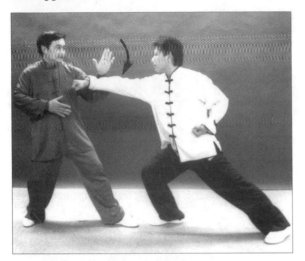

White punches to Gray's chest with his right fist. Gray intercepts with his left forearm.

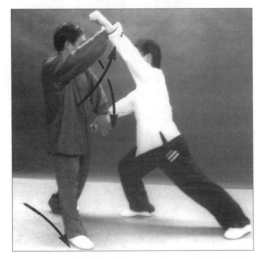

Gray pushes White's right arm down with his left hand. White follows up with a left punch to Gray's head. Gray intercepts White's left arm with his right forearm while stepping to his right with his right foot.

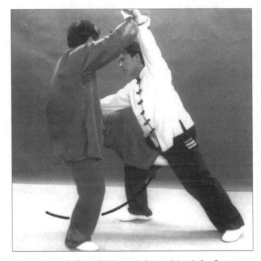

Gray then shifts all his weight to his right foot and kicks to White's groin with his left foot.

Second application

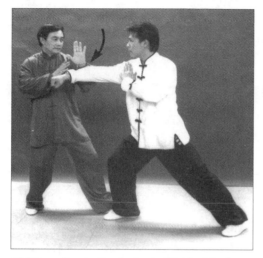

White punches to Gray's chest with his right fist. Gray intercepts with his left forearm.

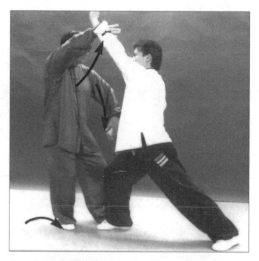

Gray moves White's right arm down to his left. White follows up with a left punch to Gray's head. Gray intercepts White's left arm with his right forearm. At the same time, Gray makes a half step forward with his right foot and moves his left foot to the side of White's right foot.

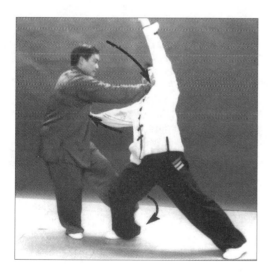

Gray then chops down to White's neck with his right palm while hooking and pulling White's knee with his left foot.

Third application

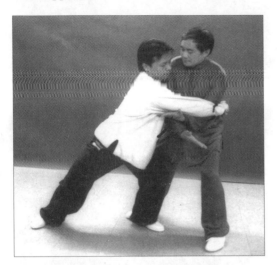

White bear-hugs Gray and attempts to lift him up.

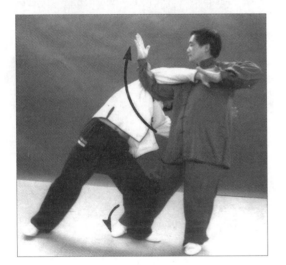

Gray pushes up on White's elbow with his left palm, lifts his right arm up, and rotates to his right to break White's hold. At the same time, Gray hooks on to White's ankle with his right foot and sweeps it to his left.

SECTION II

Posture 4: Brush Knee and Step Forward (Lou Xi Ao Bu)
Movements

Brush Knee and Step Forward, left side

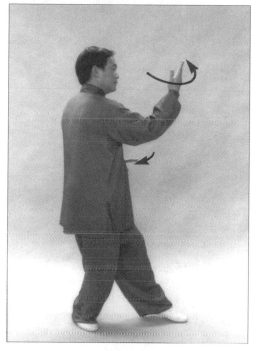

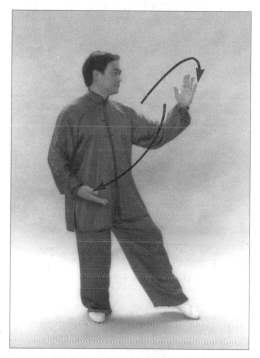

Turn your body slightly to your left while rotating your right palm to face you. (Inhale.)

Turn your body to your right while lowering your right hand down to your waist and circling your left arm up with your palm facing to your right. (Exhale.)

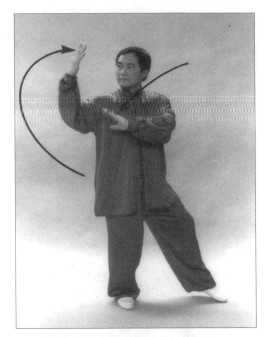

Turn your body farther to your right while lowering your left hand and circling your right hand up. Eyes look at your right palm. (Inhale.)

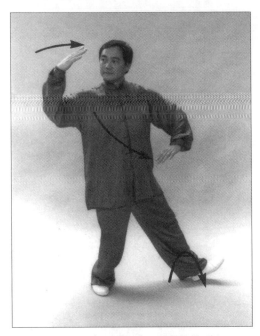

Lift up your left foot slightly and step forward while beginning to brush your left palm across your left knee, and extend your right palm forward. (Begin to exhale.)

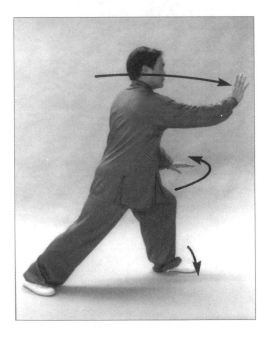

Shift your weight to your left foot into bow stance and extend your right palm forward.

Brush Knee and Step Forward, right side

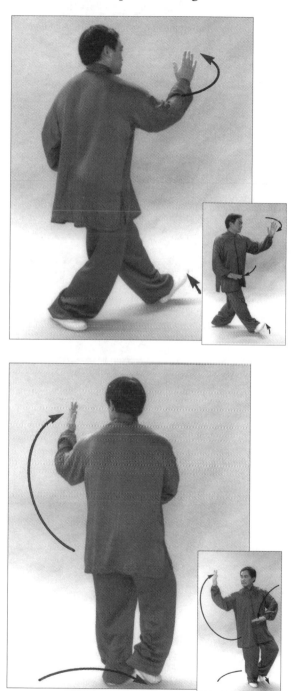

Shift your weight to your right foot. Turn your left foot outward and begin turning your body to your left while rotating your right palm inward and pulling your left palm next to your abdomen. (See mirror image. Begin to inhale.)

Bring your right foot forward next to your left while circling your left arm up to head level and begin lowering your right palm, face down. (See mirror image.)

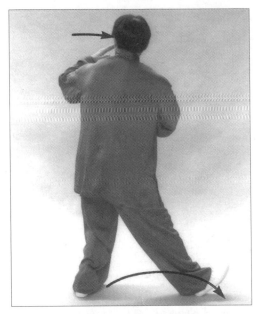

Step forward with your right foot while beginning to brush your right palm across your right knee and extend your left palm forward. (Begin to exhale.)

Shift your weight to your right foot into bow stance and extend your left palm forward.

Brush Knee and Step Forward, left side

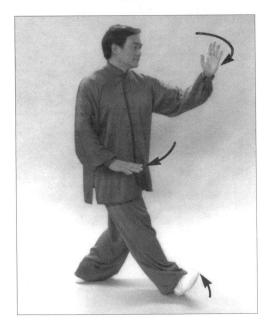

Shift your weight to your left foot. Turn your right foot outward and begin turning your body to your right while rotating your left palm inward and pulling your right palm next to your abdomen. (Begin to inhale.)

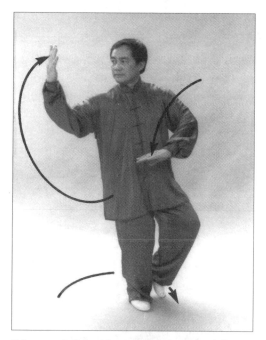

Bring your left foot forward next to your right while circling your right arm up to head level and begin lowering your left palm, face down.

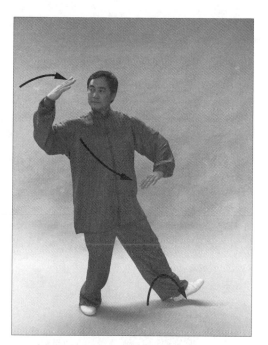

Step forward with your left foot while beginning to brush your left palm across your left knee and extend your right palm forward. (Begin to exhale.)

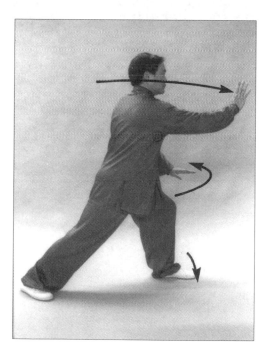

Shift your weight to your left foot into bow stance and extend your right palm forward.

Key Points

When the front hand is extended forward, maintain the body in an upright position. Do not lean forward or backward. Keep your waist and hips loose. When settling your palm, make sure your shoulders are relaxed and your elbows are dropped. As you shift your weight forward and extend your arms, imagine you are throwing a baseball; plant your back foot and feel your arms manifest the motion generated from your leg.

Brush knee and step forward means to embrace the knee and step out. Traditional long form requires that the knees be lifted before stepping forward. In the simplified sequence it is not necessary to lift the knee. *Ao bu* is a martial arts term that means opposite arm and leg forward. In this posture, it is the right arm and left leg forward or the left arm and right leg forward. The attacking arm and the front leg should be on opposite sides. When the left leg is forward, it is called a left brush knee and step forward, and vice versa.

Applications

First application

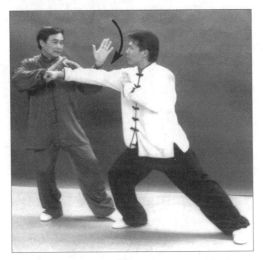

White punches to Gray's chest with his right fist. Gray intercepts with his left forearm.

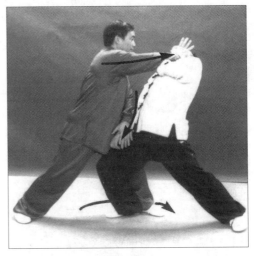

Gray then seals White's right arm down while stepping forward with his left foot and striking to White's jaw with his right palm.

Second application

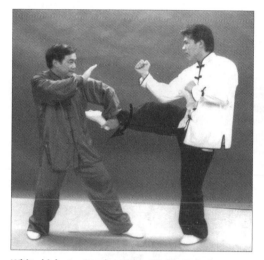

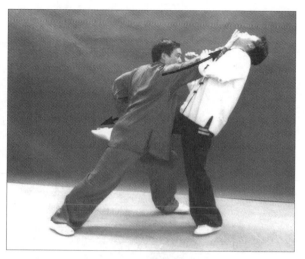

White kicks to Gray's groin with his right foot. Gray intercepts with his left hand and hooks it to his left.

Gray then steps forward with his left foot and strikes White's jaw with his right palm.

Third application

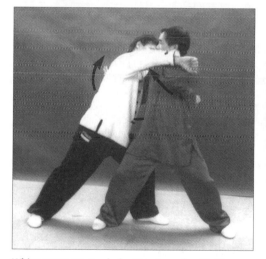

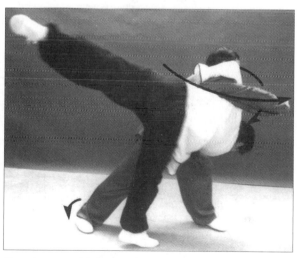

White attempts to choke Gray's neck with his arms. Gray intercepts White's right arm with his left palm and extends his right arm under White's left arm.

Gray then turns his body to his left while pulling White's right arm down with his left hand and pulling his right arm over his head and forward. This throws White forward and down.

Posture 5: Playing the Lute (Shou Hui Pipa)

Movements

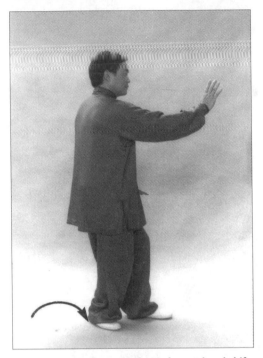

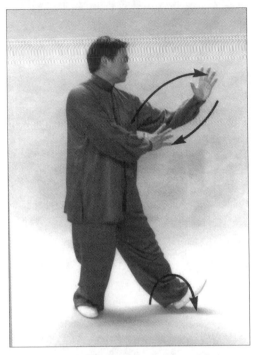

Bring your right foot a half step forward and shift your weight on it. (Inhale.)

Lift up your left foot and touch down with your heel while circling your right palm down and circling your left palm forward. Both palms face inward. (Exhale.)

Key Points

The playing the lute posture resembles a musician strumming the lute, a Chinese musical instrument. As you do this posture, check to make sure your shoulders are relaxed, your elbows are dropped, and your chest area is relaxed. When lifting your left hand, do not lift it straight up; raise it up and forward in a circular manner. When making the half step with your right foot, touch down with the ball of your foot first, and then gradually shift your weight on it. The shifting of weight and your arm movements should be completed simultaneously. Each hand makes half a circle, drawing a complete circle in front of your chest. As you finish the circle, squeeze your hands in slightly and release. Imagine you are squeezing a coiled spring and when the pressure is released, the spring pushes your hands back out.

Application

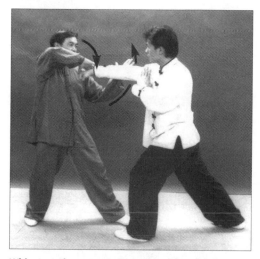

White punches to Gray's chest with his right fist. Gray intercepts with both palms, right palm on White's wrist and left palm on White's elbow.

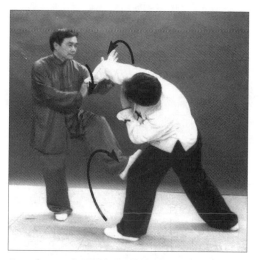

Gray then grabs hold of White's right wrist with his right hand and twists it clockwise down. At the same time, Gray pushes up on White's elbow and kicks to White's knee with his left foot.

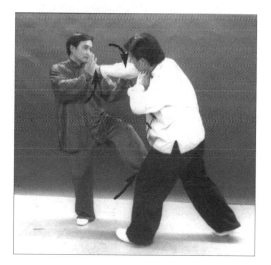

As an alternative, Gray could squeeze both palms in and break White's elbow while kicking to White's groin with his left foot.

Posture 6: Reverse Reeling Forearm (Dao Juan Gong)

Also called Repulse Monkey (Dao Nian Hou)

Movements

Reverse Reeling Forearm, right side

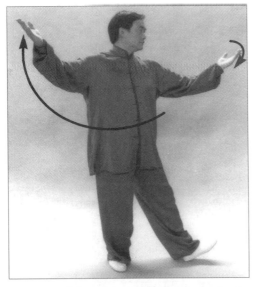

Lower your right arm as you lift it up and extend it behind you while rotating both palms up. (Begin to inhale.)

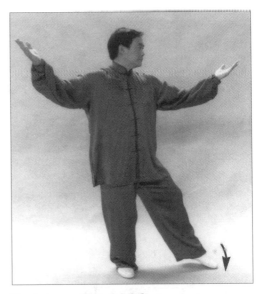

Touch down with your left foot.

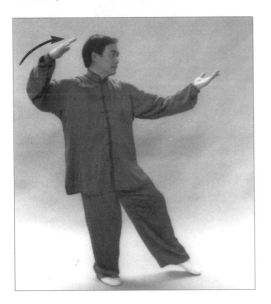

Bend your right elbow and begin stepping back with your left foot. (Begin to exhale.)

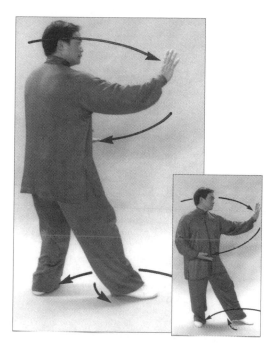

Complete stepping with your left foot behind your right foot, pivot on the balls of your feet, and turn your body toward your left while pulling your left palm next to your waist and extending your right palm forward. (See mirror image.)

Reverse Reeling Forearm, left side

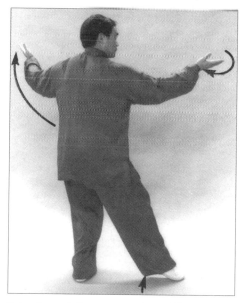

Extend your left arm out and up while rotating both palms up. (Inhale.)

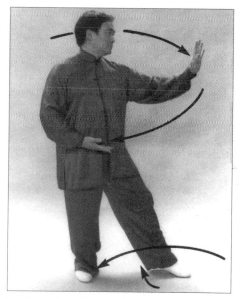

Bend your left elbow and step back with your right foot behind your left, pivot on the balls of your feet, and turn your body toward your right while pulling your right palm next to your waist and extending your left palm forward. (Exhale.)

Reverse Reeling Forearm, right side

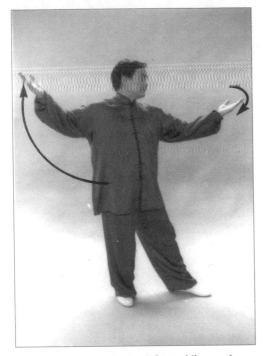 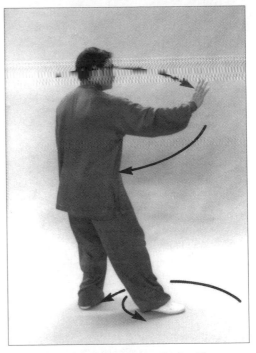

Extend your right arm out and up while rotating both palms up. (Inhale.)

Bend your right elbow and step back with your left foot behind your right, pivot on the balls of your feet, and turn your body toward your left while pulling your left palm next to your waist and extending your right palm forward. (Exhale.)

Reverse Reeling Forearm, left side

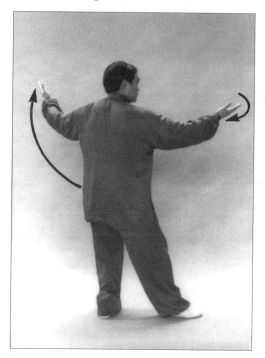

Extend your left arm out and up while rotating both palms up. (Inhale.)

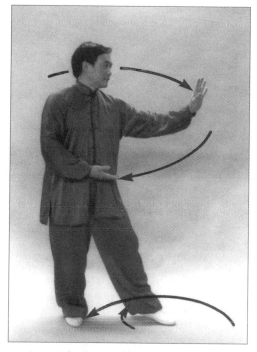

Bend your left elbow and step back with your right foot behind your left, pivot on the balls of your feet, and turn your body toward your right while pulling your right palm next to your waist and extending your left palm forward. (Exhale.)

Key Points

Do not lock the elbows when extending forward. When stepping back, touch down on the ball of your foot first, and then gradually shift your weight on it. At the same time, rotate on the ball of your front foot as you turn your body. When stepping with your right foot, step slightly to your back right corner; when stepping with your left, step slightly to your back left corner. This will prevent your feet from crossing and losing your balance. Your eyes should follow the movement of your active hand. Pay attention to your palms as they glide past each other. Imagine the palm extending forward is like a stone skipping over water. With practice you will be able to sense this skipping sensation as a magnetic repulsion caused by the energy in your palms.

Applications

First application

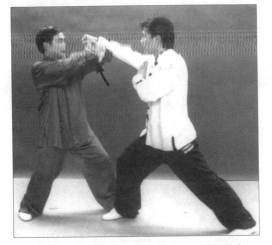

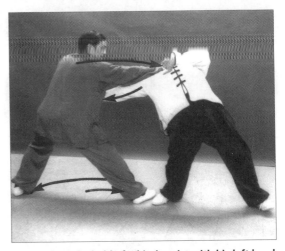

White punches to Gray's head with his right fist. Gray intercepts with his left forearm.

Gray then grabs hold of White's wrist with his left hand and pulls down as he steps back with his left foot. At the same time, Gray strikes to White's head with his right palm.

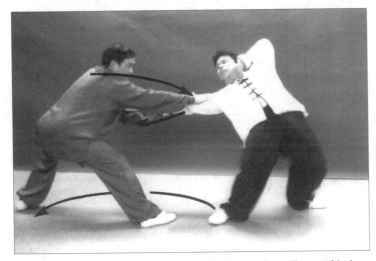

As an alternative, if the distance is too wide for a palm strike to White's head, Gray could press down on White's forearm with his right palm and drop White on the floor.

Second application

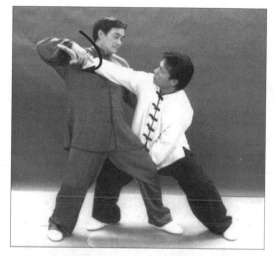

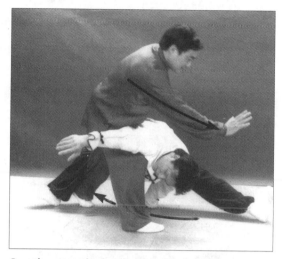

White attempts to lift up Gray's left leg by extending his right arm toward White's neck and hooking his left hand under Gray's knee. Gray hooks onto White's left wrist with his right hand and pulls down.

Gray then steps back with his left foot taking White's right leg with it, making White fall to the ground.

Third application

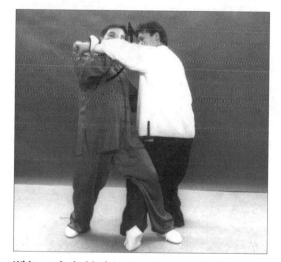

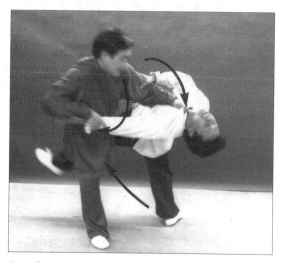

White grabs hold of Gray's left wrist with his right hand, swinging his left arm toward Gray's neck and sweeping back with his left leg on Gray's left leg, attempting to throw Gray down. Gray intercepts White's left arm with his right forearm, preventing his neck from being choked by White.

Gray then reverses the situation by grabbing hold of White's left wrist and pulling down while sweeping his left foot back, taking White's left leg off the floor. At the same time, Gray strikes forward to White's neck with his left palm.

SECTION III

Posture 7: Left Grasp the Sparrow's Tail (Zuo Lan Que Wei)

Also called Wardoff, Rollback, Press, Push (Peng, Lu, Ji, An)

Movements

Wardoff, left side

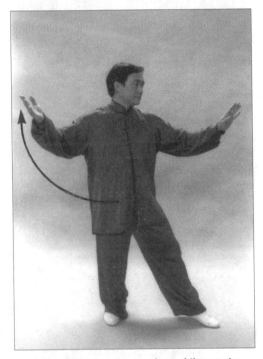

Extend your right arm out and up while rotating your right palm up. (Begin to inhale.)

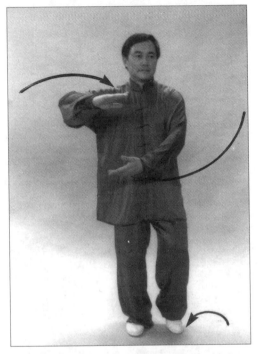

Shift all your weight to your right foot and bring your left foot next to your right while lowering your left palm and bending your right elbow until both palms face each other.

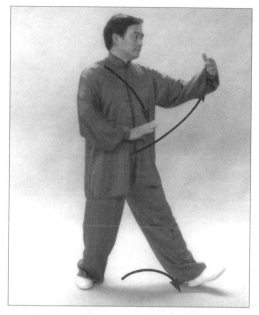

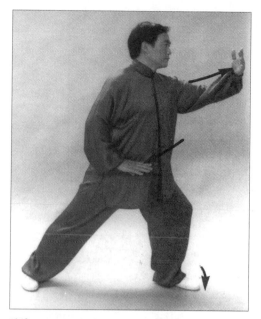

Step forward with your left foot, touching down with your heel first, while beginning to extend your left forearm forward and pulling your right palm down. (Step east. Begin to exhale.)

Shift your weight forward into a left bow stance and complete the previous arm movements. This is the completion of the left wardoff posture.

Rollback, left side

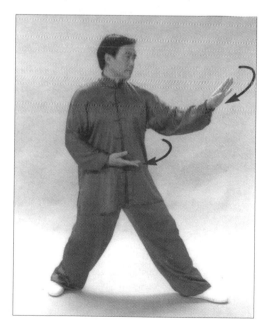

Rotate both palms clockwise, and then shift your weight back to your right foot. This is the left rollback posture. (Inhale.)

Press, left side

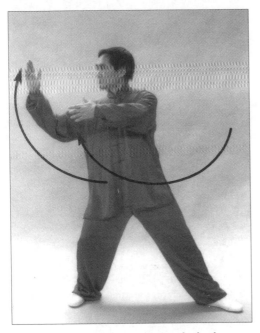

Lower both palms down and up to the back. (Exhale.)

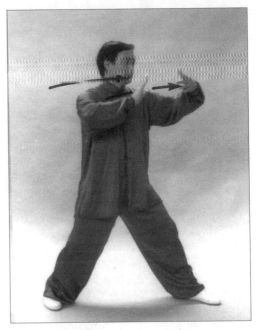

Continue the circular movements of your arms and begin extending them forward. (Inhale.)

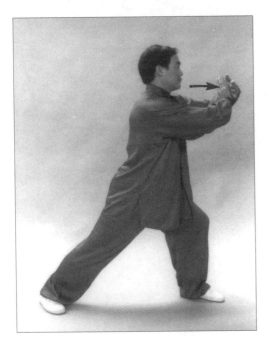

Touch your right palm to your left wrist, and extend both palms forward while shifting your weight to your left foot. This is the completion of the left press posture. (Exhale.)

Push, left side

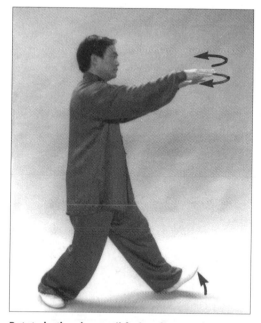

Rotate both palms until facing down and separate them while shifting your weight to your right foot. (Begin to inhale.)

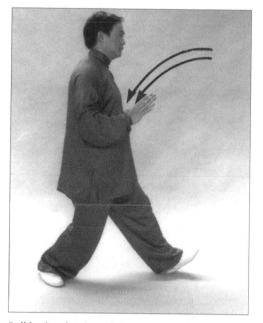

Pull both palms in and down to your abdomen.

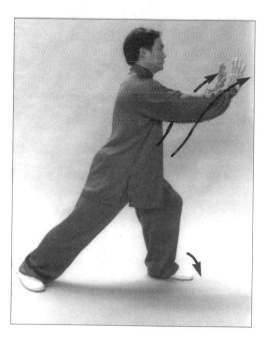

Push forward with both palms while shifting your weight to your left foot. This is the completion of the left push posture. (Exhale.)

Key Points

Grasp the sparrow's tail is referring to the grabbing of a bird's tail and playing with it. It is composed of four techniques: wardoff, rollback, press, and push, linked together and practiced as a single posture. It is a very important push hands technique. It contains the sensing, sticking, adhering, and following techniques in the taijiquan push hands applications. It requires that you maintain your center and root while being able to stick, adhere, and follow your opponent's movements, making his attack ineffective, without a solid target.

The movements are like a bop bag (a toy that is easily tipped and returns to the erect position because of the way it is weighted). When being pushed, it goes back; when the push is released, it follows the releasing force back. And when being pulled, it follows the pulling force. It goes along with the incoming force; it sticks, adheres, and follows the movements of the force. When doing the wardoff movement, imagine you are a fully inflated beach ball, filled with bounce and vitality, and firmly rooted to the ground. When doing the rollback movement, imagine you are immersing a beach ball into the water. When doing the press movement, release the force on the immersing beach ball and allow it to release itself from the water. When doing the push movement, again immerse the beach ball and then release the beach ball, allowing it to release itself from the water.

Applications

Wardoff, first application

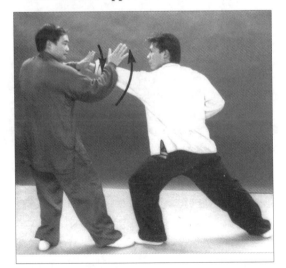 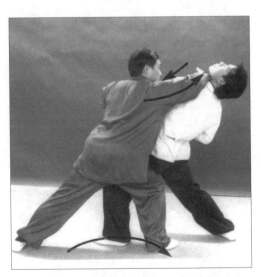

White punches to Gray's chest with his left fist. Gray intercepts with both hands and deflects White's arm to his left.

Gray grabs hold of White's left wrist with his left hand and pulls down while stepping forward with his right foot. At the same time, Gray strikes to White's neck with his right forearm.

Wardoff, second application

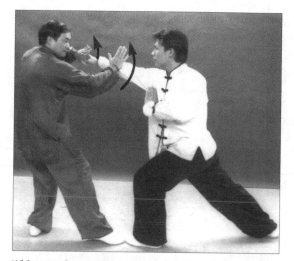

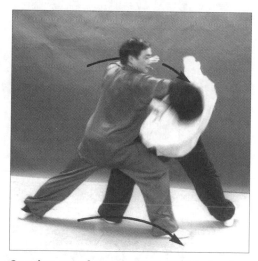

White punches to Gray's chest with his right fist. Gray intercepts with both hands and deflects White's arm to his left.

Gray then steps forward with his right foot and strikes to White's neck with his right elbow.

Rollback, first application

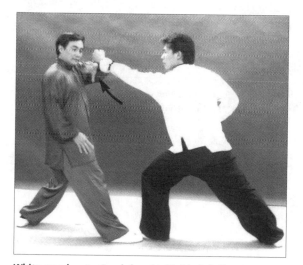

White punches to Gray's head with his left fist. Gray swings his left arm up to intercept.

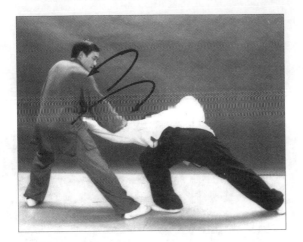

Gray then grabs hold of White's left wrist with his left hand and pulls down while extending his right arm forward and striking down on White's shoulder.

Rollback, second application

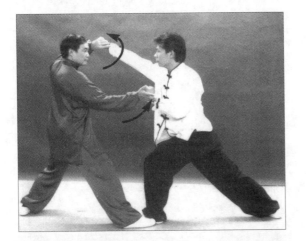

White punches to Gray's head with his right fist. Gray swings his left arm up to intercept.

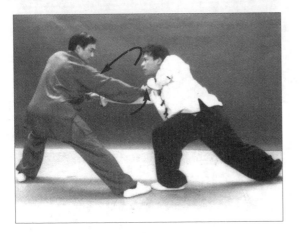

Gray then grabs hold of White's right wrist with his left hand and twists it counterclockwise down while striking his right palm forward and down on White's shoulder.

Rollback, third application

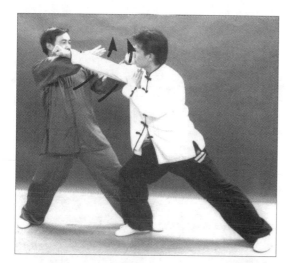

White punches to Gray's head with his right fist. Gray intercepts with both hands and deflects White's arm to his right.

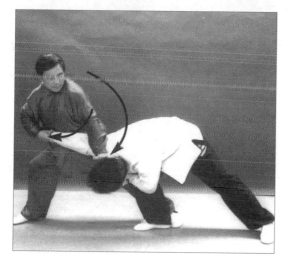

Gray then grabs hold of White's right wrist with his right hand and pulls down while striking to White's head with his left palm.

Rollback, fourth application

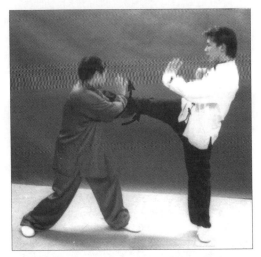

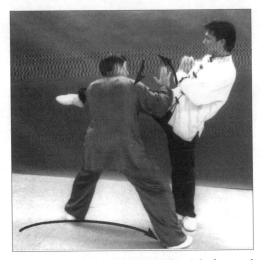

White does a roundhouse kick to Gray's body. Gray stops White's kick by intercepting White's knee with his right forearm and hooks on to White's leg with his left arm.

Gray then steps to his right with his right foot and presses down with his right forearm on White's groin area.

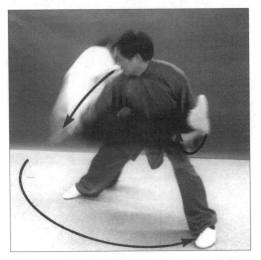

Gray turns his body to his left, pulling in with his left arm and pressing down with his right forearm to throw White to the floor.

Press, first application

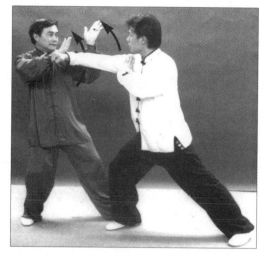

White punches to Gray's chest with his right fist. Gray intercepts with his left forearm.

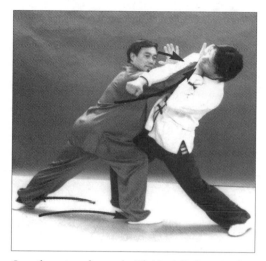

Gray then steps forward with his right foot. At the same time, Gray extends his right palm forward from under White's arm, jamming his right forearm down on White's body and pressing his left palm on White's elbow.

Press, second application

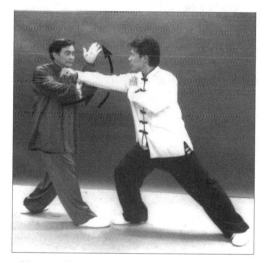

White punches to Gray's chest with his right fist. Gray intercepts with his left forearm.

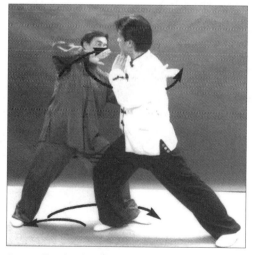

Gray coils White's right arm down to his left with his left arm. Gray then steps forward with his left foot, extends his left palm under White's armpit, and begins striking White's head with his right palm.

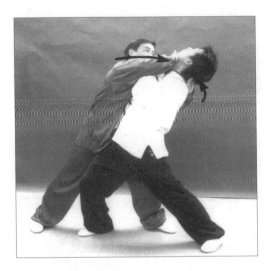

Gray completes his counterattack by grabbing the back of White's head with his left palm and striking forward and to his left, toward White's neck, with his right palm.

Push, first application

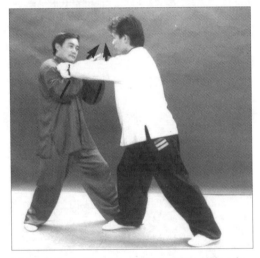

White grabs hold of Gray's shirt with both hands and attempts to pull Gray down.

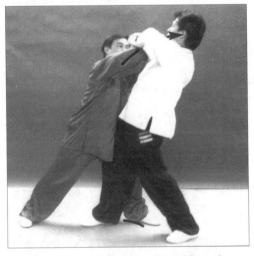

Gray steps forward and lifts White's elbows by extending both arms forward and up. Gray then strikes to White's neck with both hands.

Push, second application

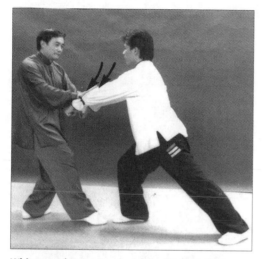 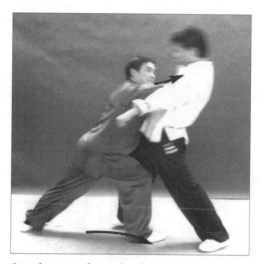

White punches to Gray's chest with both fists. Gray intercepts with both palms and leads White's punches down.

Gray then steps forward with his right foot and pushes on White's chest with both palms to drive White backward.

Posture 8: Right Grasp the Sparrow's Tail (You Lan Que Wei)

Also called Wardoff, Rollback, Press, Push (Peng, Lu, Ji, An)

Movements

Wardoff, right side

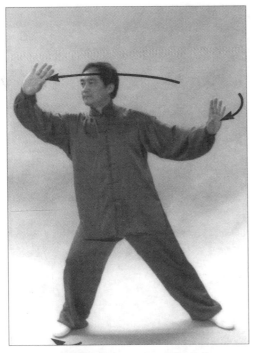

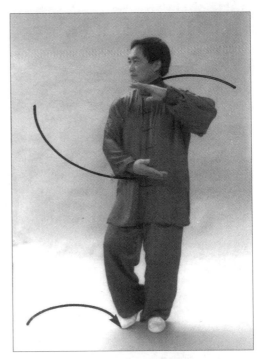

Shift your weight to your right while circling your right arm clockwise. (Begin to inhale.)

Shift your weight back to your left foot and bring your right foot next to your left foot while lowering your right palm down to abdomen level and pulling your left hand in front of your chest.

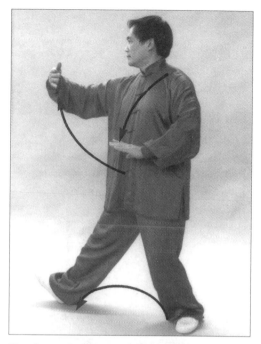

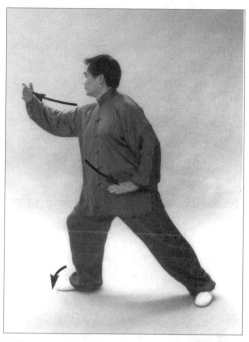

Step forward with your right foot and touch down with your heel first, while beginning to extend your right forearm forward and pulling your left palm down. (Step west. Begin to exhale.)

Shift your weight forward into a right bow stance and complete the previous arm movements. This is the completion of the right wardoff posture. (Face west.)

Rollback, right side

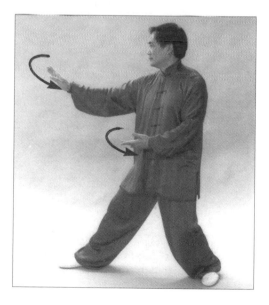

Rotate both palms counterclockwise and then shift your weight back to your left foot. This is the right rollback posture. (Inhale.)

Press, right side

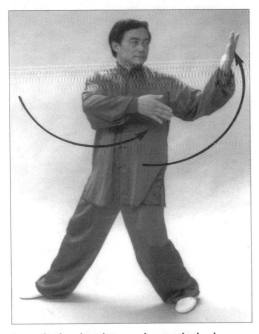

Lower both palms down and up to the back. (Exhale.)

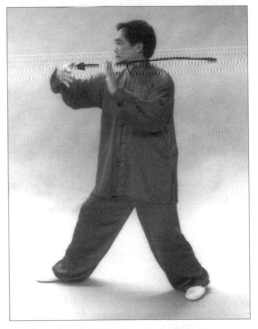

Continue the circular movements of your arms and begin extending them forward. (Inhale.)

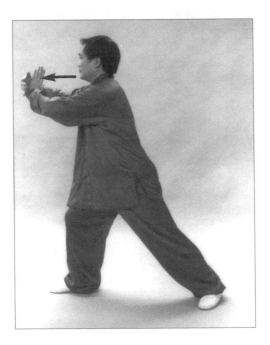

Touch your left palm to your right wrist, and extend both palms forward while shifting your weight to your right foot. This is the completion of the right press posture. (Exhale.)

Push, right side

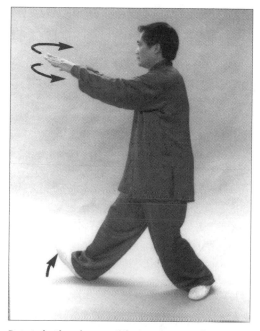

Rotate both palms until facing down and separate them while shifting your weight to your left foot. (Begin to inhale.)

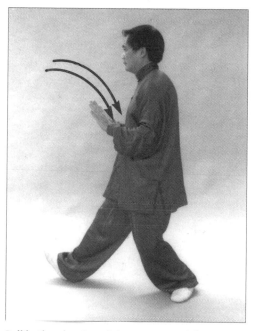

Pull both palms in and down to your abdomen.

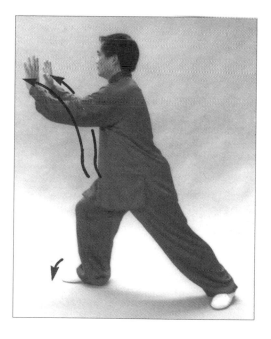

Push forward with both palms while shifting your weight to your right foot. This is the completion of the right push posture. (Exhale.)

Key Points: Same as Left Grasp Sparrow's Tail Posture

Grasp the sparrow's tail is referring to the grabbing of a bird's tail and playing with it. It is composed of four techniques: wardoff, rollback, press, and push, linked together and practiced as a single posture. It is a very important push hands technique. It contains the sensing, sticking, adhering, and following techniques in the taijiquan push hands applications. It requires that you maintain your center and root while being able to stick, adhere, and follow your opponent's movements, making his attack ineffective, without a solid target.

The movements are like a bop bag (a toy that is easily tipped and returns to the erect position because of the way it is weighted). When being pushed, it goes back; when the push is released, it follows the releasing force back. And when being pulled, it follows the pulling force. It goes along with the incoming force; it sticks, adheres, and follows the movements of the force. When doing the wardoff movement, imagine that you are a fully inflated beach ball, filled with "bounce" and vitality and firmly rooted to the ground. When doing the rollback movement, imagine that you are immersing a beach ball into the water. When doing the press movement, release the force on the immersing beach ball and allow it to release itself from the water. When doing the push movement, again immerse the beach ball and then release the beach ball, allowing it to release itself from the water.

Applications

Wardoff, first application

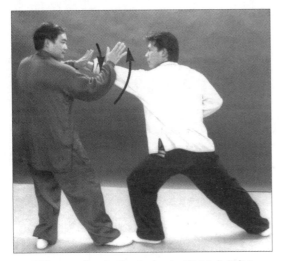

White punches to Gray's chest with his left fist. Gray intercepts with both hands and deflects White's arm to his left.

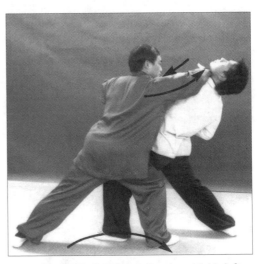

Gray grabs hold of White's left wrist with his left hand and pulls down while stepping forward with his right foot. At the same time, Gray strikes to White's neck with his right forearm.

Wardoff, second application

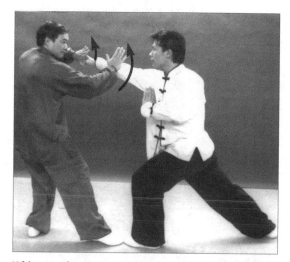

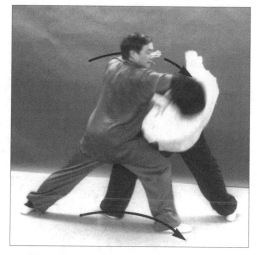

White punches to Gray's chest with his right fist. Gray intercepts with both hands and deflects White's arm to his left.

Gray then steps forward with his right foot and strikes to White's neck with his right elbow.

Rollback, first application

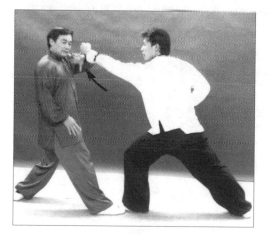

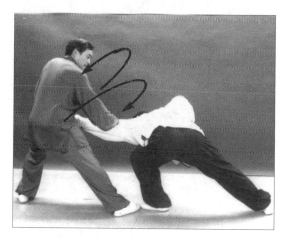

White punches to Gray's head with his left fist. Gray swings his left arm up to intercept.

Gray then grabs hold of White's left wrist with his left hand and pulls down while extending his right arm forward and striking down on White's shoulder.

Rollback, second application

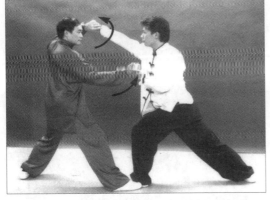

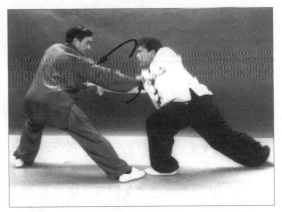

White punches to Gray's head with his right fist. Gray swings his left arm up to intercept.

Gray then grabs hold of White's right wrist with his left hand and twists it counterclockwise down, while striking his right palm forward and down on White's shoulder.

Rollback, third application

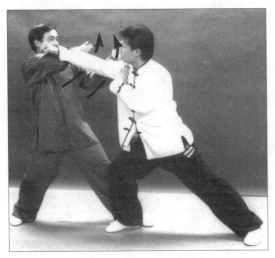

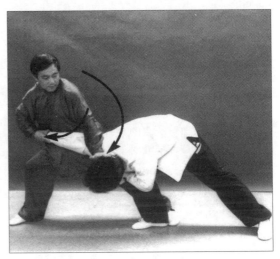

White punches to Gray's head with his right fist. Gray intercepts with both hands and deflects White's arm to his right.

Gray then grabs hold of White's right wrist with his right hand and pulls down while striking to White's head with his left palm.

Rollback, fourth application

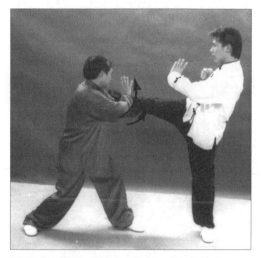

White does a roundhouse kick to Gray's body. Gray stops White's kick by intercepting White's knee with his right forearm and hooks on to White's leg with his left arm.

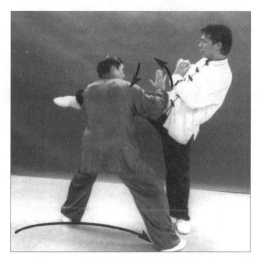

Gray then steps to his right with his right foot and presses down with his right forearm on White's groin area.

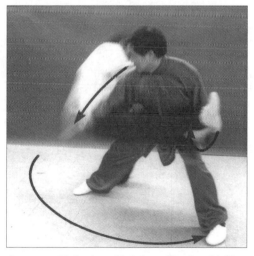

Gray turns his body to his left, pulling in with his left arm and pressing down with his right forearm to throw White to the floor.

Press, first application

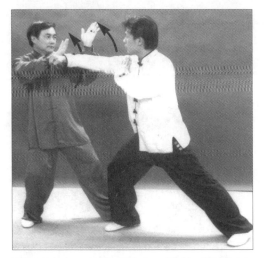

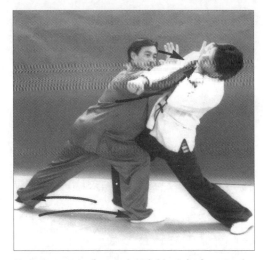

White punches to Gray's chest with his right fist. Gray intercepts with his left forearm.

Gray then steps forward with his right foot. At the same time, Gray extends his right palm forward from under White's arm, jamming his right forearm down on White's body and pressing his left palm on White's elbow.

Press, second application

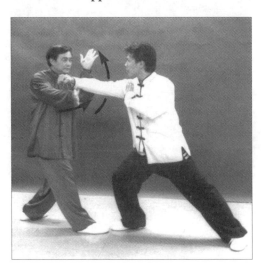

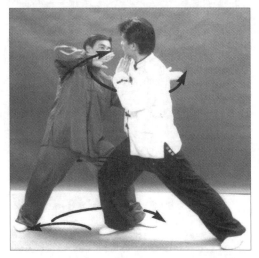

White punches to Gray's chest with his right fist. Gray intercepts with his left forearm.

Gray coils White's right arm down to his left, with his left arm. Gray then steps forward with his left foot, extends his left palm under White's armpit, and begins striking White's head with his right palm.

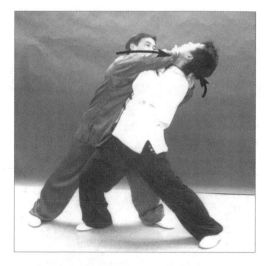

Gray completes his counterattack by grabbing the back of White's head with his left palm and striking forward and to his left, toward White's neck, with his right palm.

Push, first application

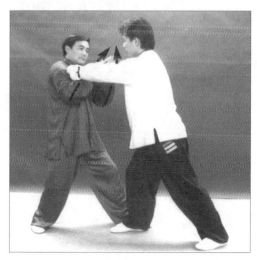

White grabs hold of Gray's shirt with both hands and attempts to pull Gray down.

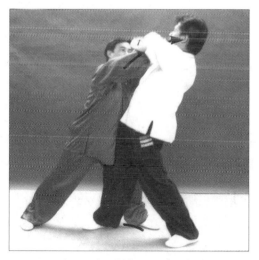

Gray steps forward and lifts up White's elbows by extending both arms forward and up. Gray then strikes to White's neck with both hands.

Push, second application

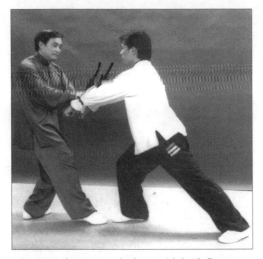 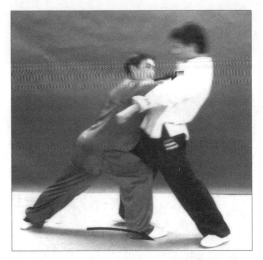

White punches to Gray's chest with both fists. Gray intercepts with both palms and leads White's punches down.

Gray then steps forward with his right foot and pushes on White's chest with both palms to drive White backward.

SECTION IV

Posture 9: Single Whip (Dan Bian)

Movements

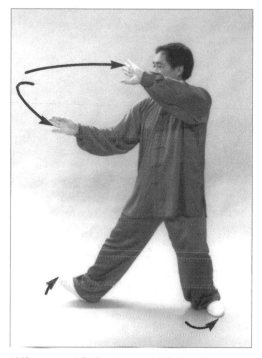

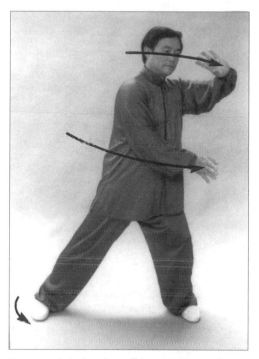

Shift your weight back to your left foot. Rotate palms until they both face out, and begin to circle both arms to your left. (Begin to inhale.)

Turn your right foot in until it points forward while continuing to circle your arms to your left.

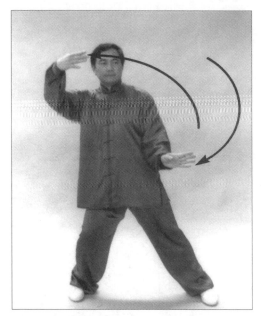

Shift your weight back to your right foot while circling your left hand down and circling your right palm up across your head. (Begin to exhale.)

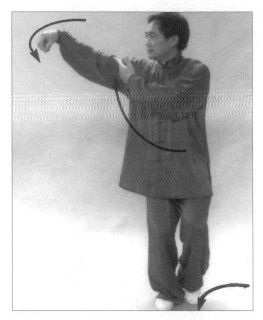

Bring your left foot next to your right foot while hooking your right hand out to your back right corner and bringing your left palm next to your right shoulder.

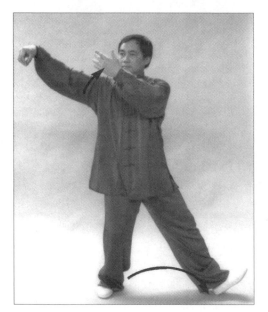

Step to your left with your left foot, and begin to rotate and extend your left palm forward. (Inhale.)

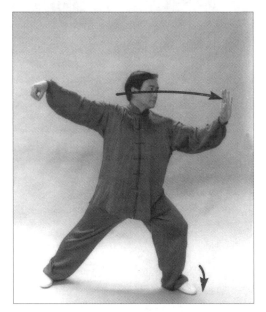

Shift your weight to your left foot and complete your left palm rotation and extension forward. (Exhale. Face east.)

Key Points

Single whip is referring to the motion of a whip snapping forward. When executing this posture, keep your body erect and waist relaxed. When you complete this posture, keep your right elbow slightly bent, align your left elbow up with your left knee, and keep both shoulders relaxed. When rotating and extending your left hand, it should be completed with the turning of your body. As you push down with your right foot, your waist turns and guides the motion that is generated by your foot, and extends your left hand out, resembling the motion of a whip.

Applications

First application

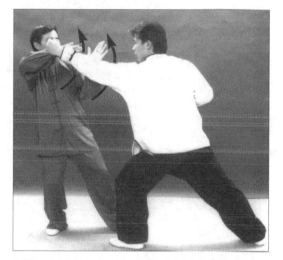

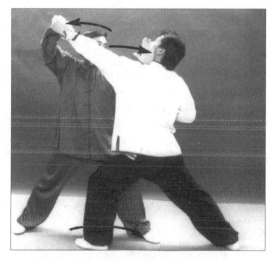

White punches to Gray's head with his left fist. Gray intercepts with both palms.

Gray then grabs hold of White's left wrist with his right hand and pulls back and up. At the same time, Gray steps forward with his left foot and chops to White's neck with the edge of his left palm.

Second application

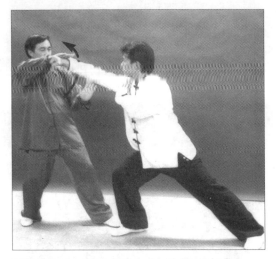

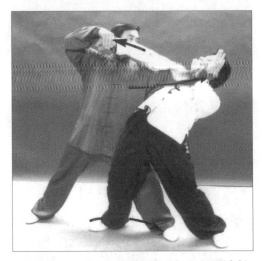

White punches to Gray's head with his right fist. Gray intercepts with his right palm.

Gray then grabs hold of White's right wrist with his right hand and pulls back and up. At the same time, Gray steps forward with his left foot and strikes his left palm toward White's collarbone. Notice White's arm is locked on top of Gray's left arm.

Posture 10: Wave Hands Like Clouds (Yun Shou)

Movements

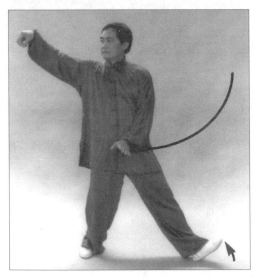

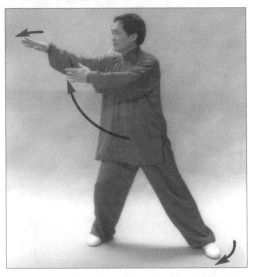

Lower your left hand and shift your weight to your right foot. Lift up the ball of your foot. (Begin to inhale.)

Turn your left foot in until it points forward while beginning to circle your left palm up and open your right palm.

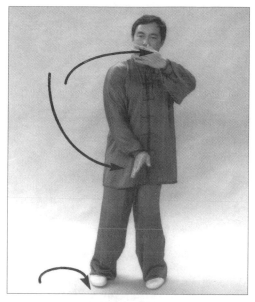

Continue circling your left palm up and across
your face while lowering your right hand and
moving your right foot closer to your left foot.
(Begin to exhale.)

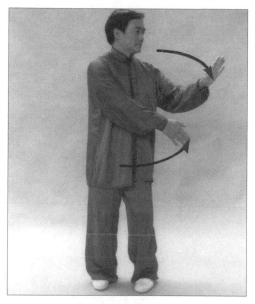

Continue with the previous palm movements,
lowering your left palm and lifting your right
palm.

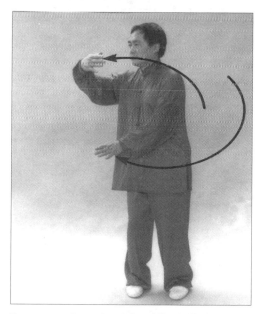

Turn your waist to the right while circling your
right palm up and across your face and lowering
your left palm.

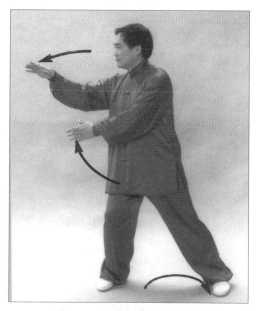

Step to your left with your left foot while
extending your right palm to the side, palm down,
and begin lifting your left palm up. (Begin to
inhale.)

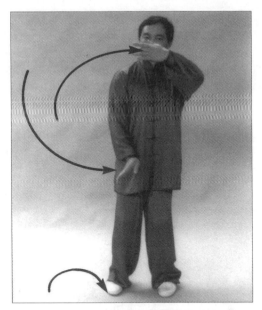

Continue circling your left palm up and across your face while lowering your right hand and moving your right foot closer to your left foot.

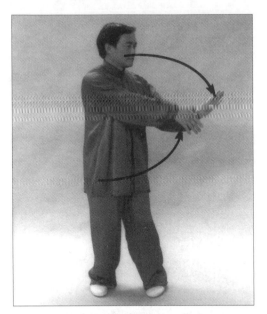

Continue with the previous palm movements, lowering your left palm and lifting your right palm. (Begin to exhale.)

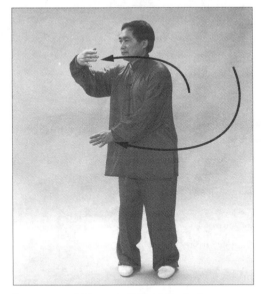

Turn your waist to your right while circling your right palm up and across your face and lowering your left palm.

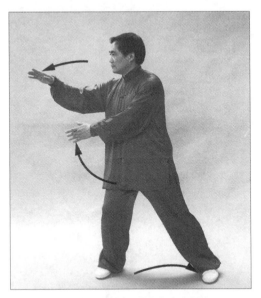

Step to your left with your left foot while extending your right palm to the side, palm down, and begin lifting up your left palm. (Begin to inhale.)

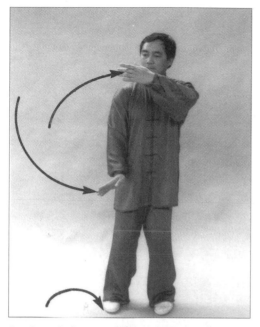

Continue circling your left palm up and across your face while lowering your right hand and moving your right foot closer to your left foot.

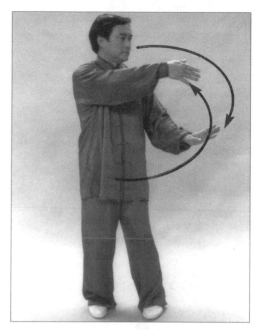

Continue with the previous palm movements, lowering your left palm and lifting your right palm. (Begin to exhale.)

Key Points

Wave hands like clouds is referring to the movement of the arms, as though they were clouds moving past each other—not touching and moving in unison. As the lower hand moves up, it is like a scooping movement. Use your waist to direct the movements of your upper body. Keep your waist and hips relaxed. Maintain one height as you step. Your arms should follow the movements of your waist. When moving your upper body, make sure your feet are well rooted. Touch down on the ball of your foot before solidifying your stance.

Each hand draws a circle overlapping in front of your body. To make learning easier, start by standing in a horse stance, and then break the movements down into three distinct pieces: (1) Hands up and down, (2) Turn body, and (3) Step.

For example,

1.   With your feet apart in a horse stance, as your right hand moves down your left moves up.

2.   Turn your body to your left and shift your weight to your left foot.

3.   Step with your right foot, bringing it closer to your left one.

To continue,

1. With your feet apart in a horse stance, move your left hand down as your right hand moves up.
2. Turn your body to your right and shift your weight to your right foot.
3. Step with your left foot, bringing it closer to your right one.

Once you have the up and down, turn, and step movements coordinated, blend them together into one fluid motion.

Applications

First application

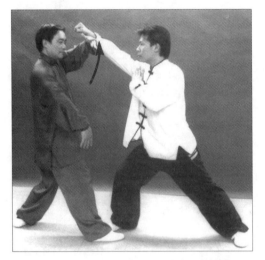

White punches to Gray's head with his right fist. Gray intercepts by lifting up his left forearm.

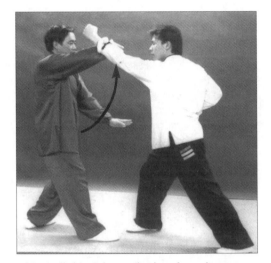

White pulls his right arm back and punches to Gray's head with his left fist. Gray intercepts by lifting up his right forearm.

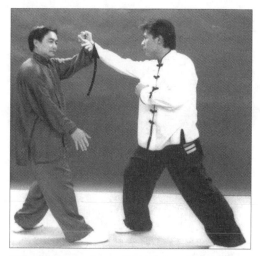

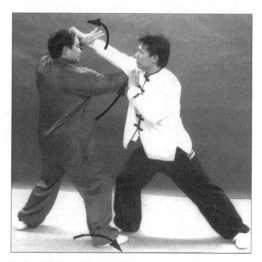

White pulls his left arm back and again punches to Gray's head with his right fist. Gray lifts his left forearm again to intercept.

Before White pulls his right arm back, Gray grabs hold of White's right wrist while lifting up White's upper arm with his right forearm.

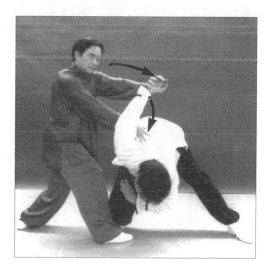

Gray then pushes White's wrist forward and hooks his right hand on White's biceps while turning his body to his right to lock White's arm.

Second application

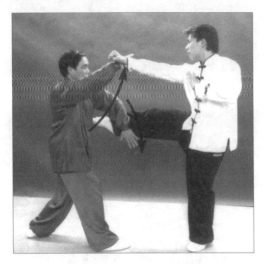

White kicks to Gray's groin with his right foot and punches to Gray's head with his right fist simultaneously. Gray intercepts White's kick by lowering his left forearm and intercepts White's arm by lifting with his right forearm.

Third application

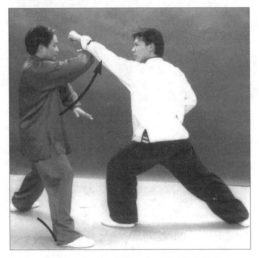

White punches to Gray's head with his left fist. White intercepts by lifting his right forearm while stepping to his right with his right foot.

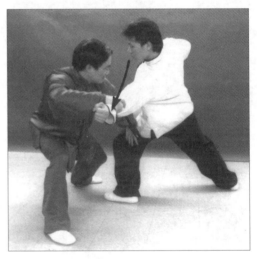

Gray then grabs hold of White's left wrist and pulls down while pressing his left palm on White's left knee, dropping White to the floor.

Posture 11: Single Whip (Dan Bian)

Movements

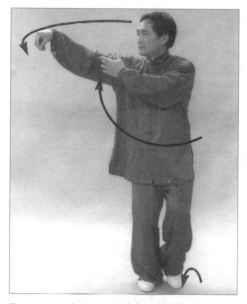

Turn your waist to your right while hooking your right hand to your back right corner, and bring your left palm next to your right shoulder.

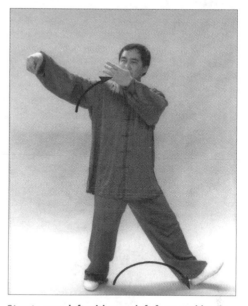

Step to your left with your left foot, and begin to rotate and extend your left palm forward. (Inhale.)

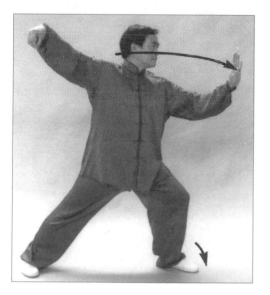

Shift your weight to your left foot and complete your left palm rotation and extension forward. (Exhale.)

SECTION V

Posture 12: High Pat on Horse (Gao Tan Ma)

Movements

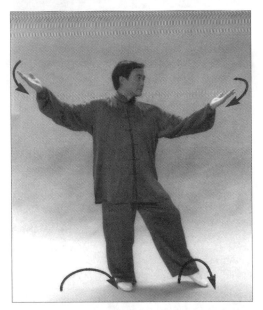

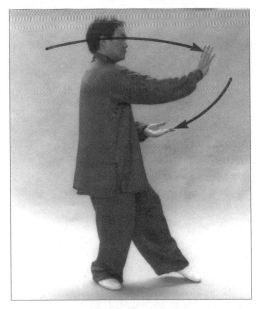

Bring your right foot a half step forward and shift all your weight on it while rotating both palms up. (Inhale.)

Bend your right elbow and extend your right palm forward while pulling your left palm next to your waist. (Exhale.)

Key Points

High pat on horse is referring to a rider gauging the height of the horse's back before mounting. Keep your body naturally erect and your shoulders relaxed. Drop both of your elbows slightly. When making the half step, maintain one height.

Application

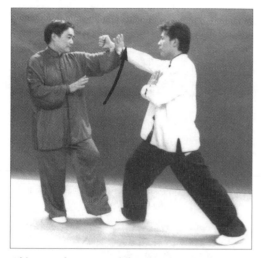

White punches to Gray's head with his right fist. Gray intercepts by lifting his left forearm.

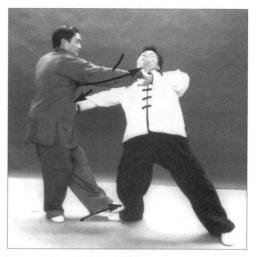

Gray then grabs hold of White's right wrist with his left hand and pulls it back and down. At the same time, Gray kicks to White's shin with his left foot and strikes to White's neck with the edge of his right palm.

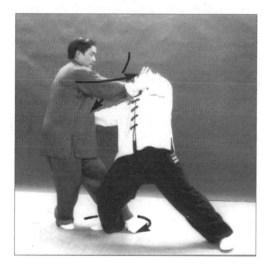

As an alternative, Gray could sweep his left foot across White's right foot while striking with his right palm on White's neck.

Posture 13: Right Heel Kick (You Deng Jiao)

Movements

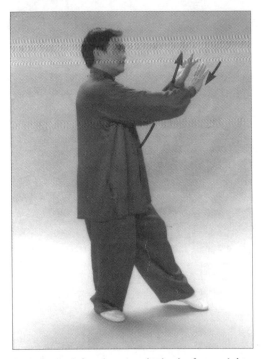

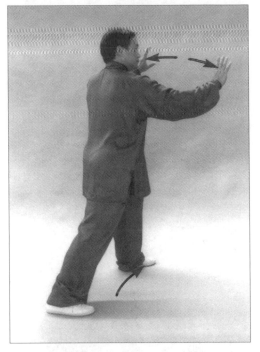

Extend your left palm over the back of your right hand. (Begin to inhale.)

Step to your left corner with your left foot and shift your weight on it while separating and beginning to lower both palms. The left palm rotates until it faces forward. (Step northeast.)

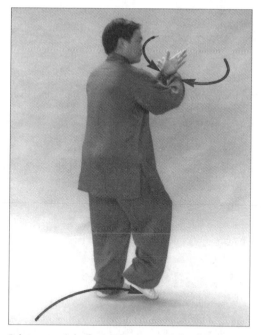

Bring your right foot next to your left while circling both palms down, then up, until your arms are crossed, with both palms facing you, right palm on the outside.

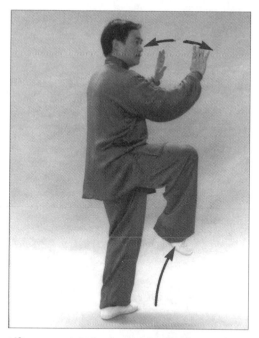

Lift up your right foot, rotate both palms until they face forward, and begin to separate your palms to the sides. (Begin to exhale.)

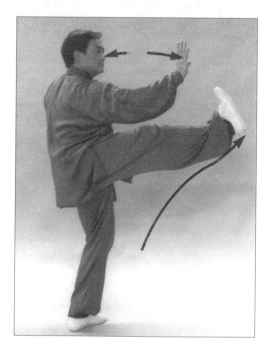

Extend your right leg to your upper right corner while extending your right palm in the same direction, and lift your palm to the left. (Face southeast.)

Key Points

Heel kick refers to kicking an opponent's body with your heel. Stabilize your body. Do not lean forward or backward. Your wrists should be at the same height as your shoulders when you separate your hands. When kicking with your right heel, bend your left knee slightly and pull your right toes up slightly. The arm extension and the kick should be executed together. Your right arm and right leg should be aligned in the same vertical plane. When pulling your hands apart, imagine you are pulling your living room curtains open, allowing the sun's energy to fill your body.

Applications

First application

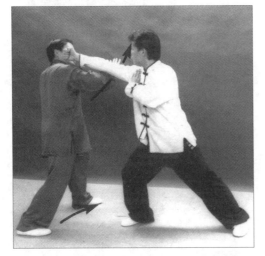

White punches to Gray's head with his right fist. Gray sidesteps to his left with his left foot while lifting his right forearm to intercept White's punch.

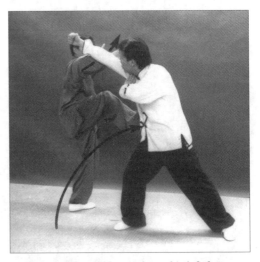

Gray then shifts all his weight on his left foot and kicks to White's ribs with the heel of his right foot.

Second application

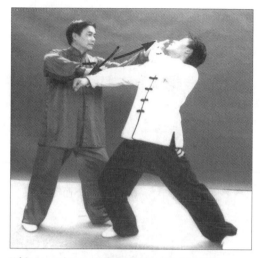

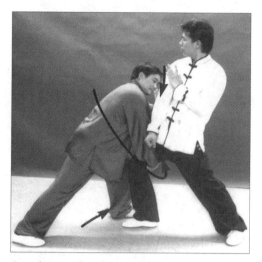

White punches to Gray's chest with his right fist. Gray intercepts with his right palm, leading White's arm down, while spearing to White's neck with his left hand.

Gray then reaches down with both hands to White's thigh and attempts to throw White down.

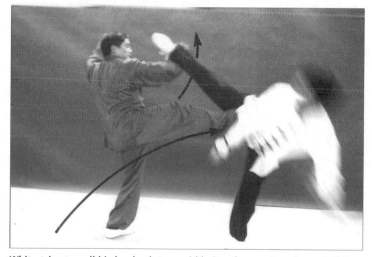

White tries to pull his leg back to avoid being thrown. Gray keeps holding on to White's leg, lifting it up and heel kicking to White's groin.

Posture 14: Strike to Ears with Both Fists (Shuang Feng Guan Er)

Movements

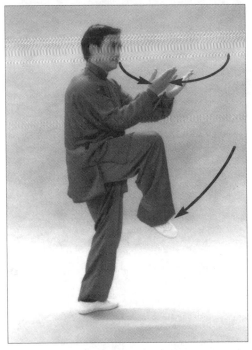

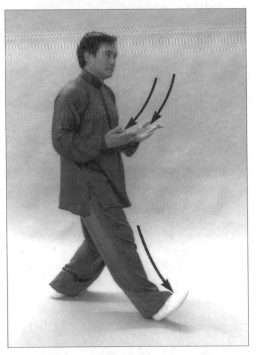

Pull your right leg back and bring both palms together until your palms are facing you. (Begin to inhale.)

Step down to your front right corner while lowering your palms next to your abdomen.

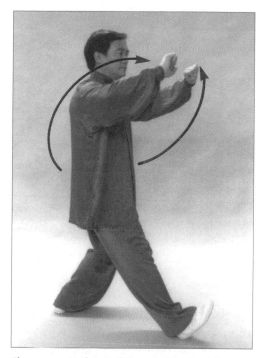

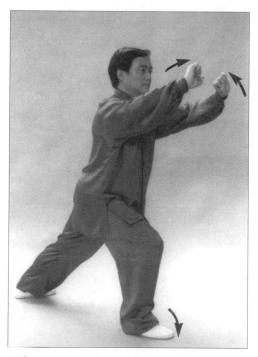

Change your palms to fists and circle both fists to your sides and up. Palms of your fists face forward. (Begin to exhale.)

Shift your weight forward to your right foot and bring your fists closer together. (Face southeast.)

Key Points

When stepping down with your right foot, bend your left knee slightly and place your right foot down gently. As you extend your fist forward, imagine you are doing the breaststroke. As you kick the water with your feet, a wavelike motion extends through your body and out to your fists. Be careful to not extend your right knee over your right toes and put too much tension on your right knee.

Application

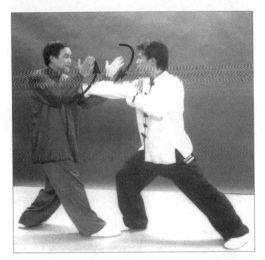

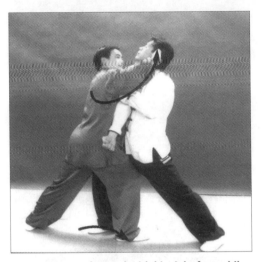

White punches to Gray's chest with his right fist. Gray intercepts with his left forearm and locks White's arm by squeezing both forearms inward.

Gray then steps forward with his right foot while sealing White's right arm down with his left palm. At the same time, Gray swings toward White's temple with a right fist.

Posture 15: Turn Body and Left Heel Kick (Zhuan Shen Zuo Deng Jiao)

Movements

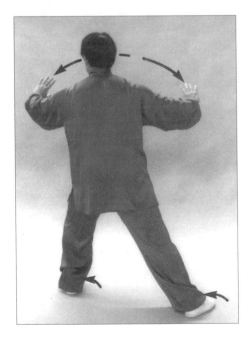

Turn your right foot in and left foot out as you turn to your left. Shift your weight to your left foot. Open your fists and separate your palms to your sides. (Begin to inhale.)

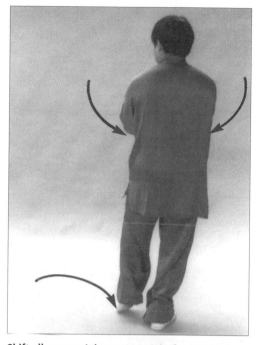

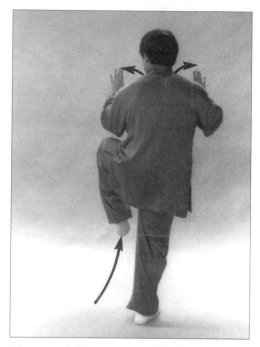

Shift all your weight on your right foot and bring your left foot next to your right while circling both palms down until they cross and the palms face you, left palm on the outside. (Similar to palm movements in posture 13.)

Lift up your left foot, rotate both palms until they face forward, and begin to separate your palms to the sides. (Begin to exhale.)

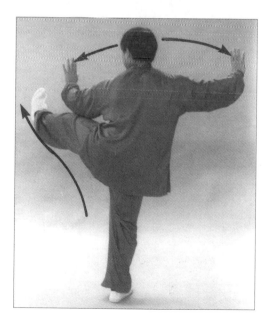

Extend your left leg to your upper left corner while extending your left palm in the same direction and right palm to your right. (Kick northwest.)

SECTION VI

Posture 16: Left Lower Body Then Stand on One Leg (Zuo Xia Shi Du Li)

Movements

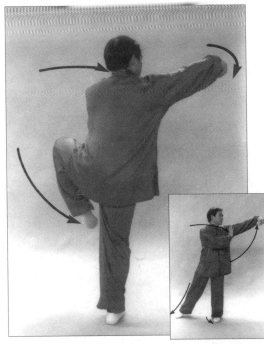

Form a hook with your right hand while pulling your left foot in and bringing your left palm next to your right shoulder. (See mirror image of hand form. Begin to inhale.)

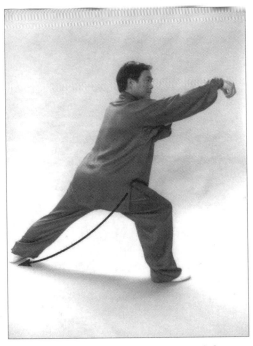

Bend your right leg and step out to your left. (Step west.)

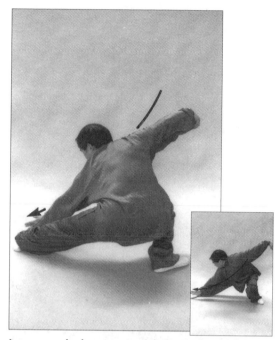

Lower your body over your right leg and extend your left palm along the inside edge of your left leg, out to your foot. (See mirror image.)

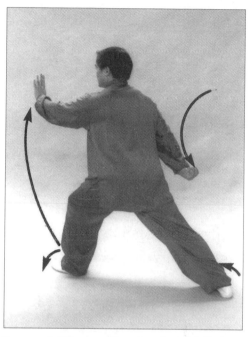

Turn your left foot until it points forward. Shift your weight forward into left bow stance while lifting your left palm up and forward and lowering your right hand behind you in a hook position, pointing up. (Face west. Begin to exhale.)

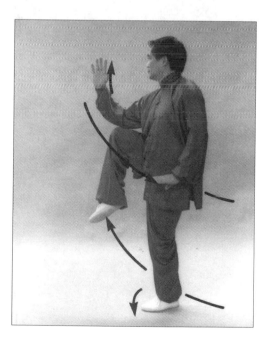

Turn your left foot out and stand up on it while lowering your left palm. At the same time, open your right hand and spear up.

Key Points

This posture is made up of two parts. The original names for this posture were snake creeps down and golden rooster stands on one leg. Snake creeps down, or the lowering of the body, is a defensive move to avoid an opponent's high attack. Golden rooster stands on one leg, or standing on one leg, is an attacking move that sets up for a kick. Keep your upper body erect. The standing leg should be slightly bent. When lifting your right leg, let your foot relax naturally. When moving your leg up, imagine your hand is lifting your leg, as though you were moving the leg of a puppet with your hand. When lowering your body, it is not necessary to go as low as is shown in the photographs. As you lower your body, make sure you bend your knee in the same direction as your foot.

Applications

Lower Body, first application

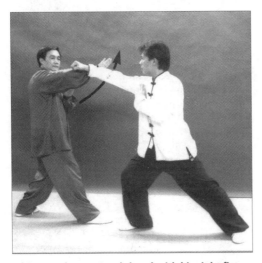
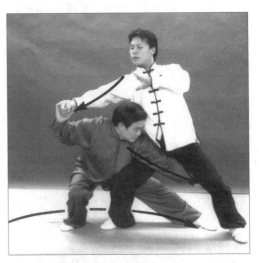

White punches to Gray's head with his right fist. Gray intercepts by circling his right forearm up.

Gray then grabs hold of White's right wrist with his right hand while stepping forward with his left foot and lowering his body. At the same time, Gray extends his left palm behind White's knee, striking White's groin along the way.

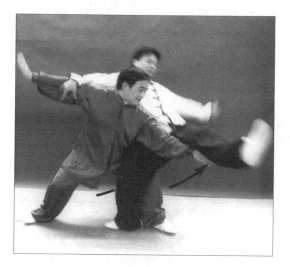

Gray continues his counterattack by shifting his weight forward, lifting up White's right leg by pressing his left thigh on White's leg while lifting up White's left leg with his left hand, dropping White to the floor.

Stand on One Leg, first application

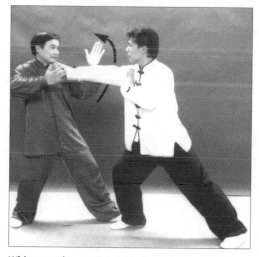

White punches to Gray's chest with his right fist. Gray intercepts with his left forearm.

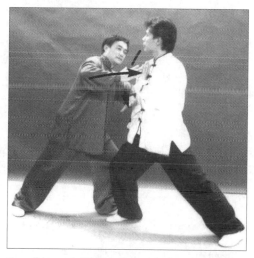

Gray then seals White's right arm down and shifts his weight forward to his left leg while spearing his right hand up toward White's neck.

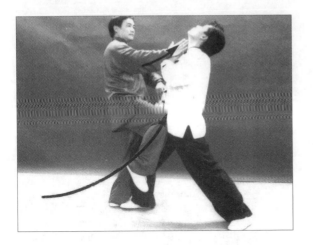

Gray continues his counterattack by kicking to White's groin by lifting his right knee, and completing his strike to White's neck with his right spear hand.

Stand on One Leg, second application

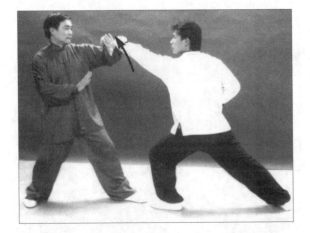

White punches to Gray's head with his left fist. Gray intercepts by circling his left forearm up.

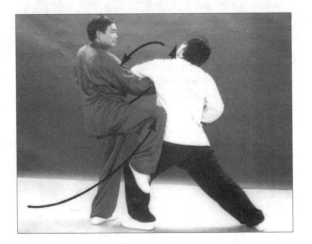

Gray then grabs hold of White's left wrist with his left hand while kicking to White's kidney area with his right knee, and striking to White's neck by spearing his right hand up from under White's left arm.

Posture 17: Right Lower Body Then Stand on One Leg (You Xia Shi Du Li)
Movements

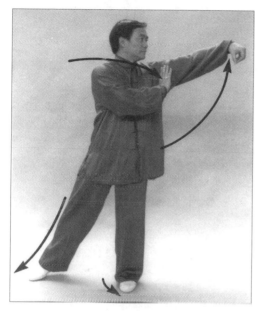

Put your right foot down in front of you. Form a hook with your left hand, and then lift and extend it backward while placing your right palm next to your left shoulder. Turn your left foot out to get ready for the next move. (Begin to inhale.)

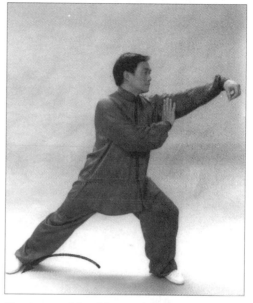

Step to your right with your right foot and bend your left knee. (Step west.)

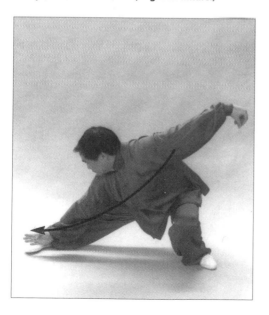

Lower your body over your left leg and extend your right palm along the inside edge of your right leg, out to your foot.

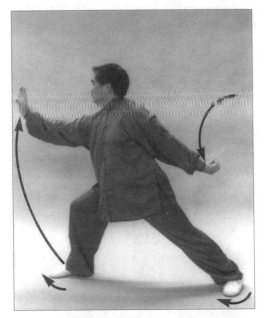

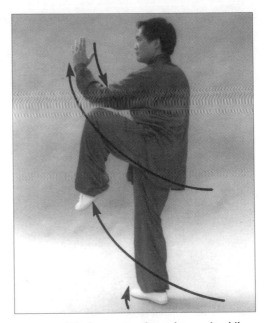

Turn your right foot until it points forward. Shift your weight forward into right bow stance while lifting your right palm and lowering your left hand behind you in a hook position, pointing up. (Face west. Begin to exhale.)

Turn your right foot out and stand up on it while lowering your right palm. At the same time, open your left hand and spear up.

SECTION VII

Posture 18: Shuttle Back and Forth (Chuan Suo)

Movements

Shuttle Back and Forth, right side

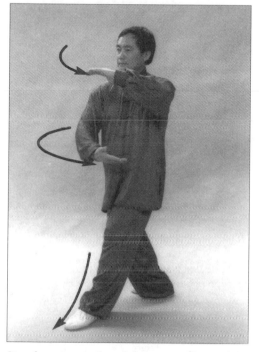 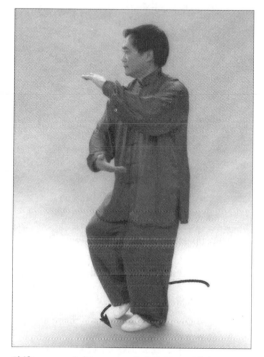

Step down to your front left corner with your left foot. Bring your right palm next to your stomach, palm faces up, and lower your left palm next to your chest, palm faces down. (**Step southwest. Begin to inhale.**)

Shift your weight on your left foot and bring your right foot next to your left. (**Face southwest.**)

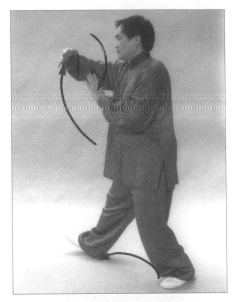

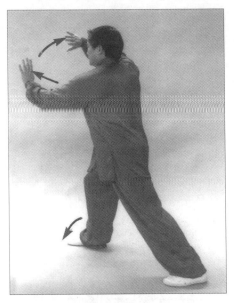

Step to your front right corner with your right foot, begin to raise your right forearm, and extend your left palm. Left elbow should be down. (Step northwest. Begin to exhale.)

Shift your weight forward into right bow stance, raise your right forearm to your head level, and extend your left palm in front of you. (Face northwest.)

Shuttle Back and Forth, left side

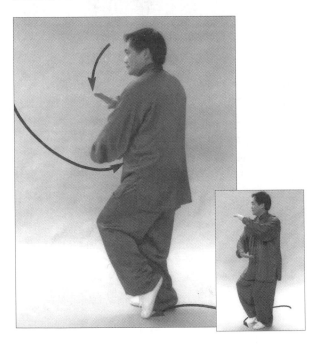

First, shift your weight back to your left foot and turn your right foot out slightly. Then shift all your weight to your right foot and bring your left foot next to your right. Bring your left palm down next to your stomach, palm facing up, and lower your right palm next to your chest, palm facing down. (See mirror image. Inhale.)

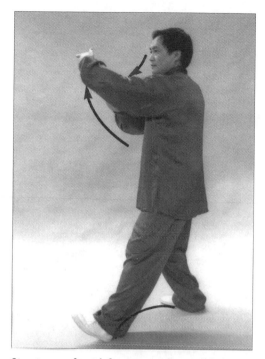

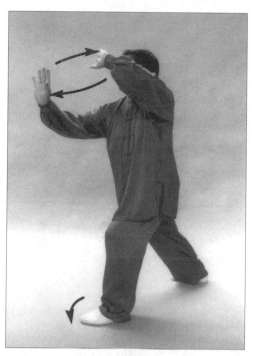

Step to your front left corner with your left foot, begin to raise your left arm, and extend your right palm. Right elbow should be down. (Step southwest. Begin to exhale.)

Shift your weight forward into left bow stance, raise your left forearm to your head level, and extend your right palm in front of you. (Face southwest.)

Key Points

Shuttle back and forth is referring to the weaver's shuttle, moving back and forth. This posture's name was used to describe the fast movements that were used to defend against multiple opponents from multiple directions. As you do this posture, imagine that you are an expert weaver, weaving the shuttle under and over the threads, creating an intricate pattern.

Application

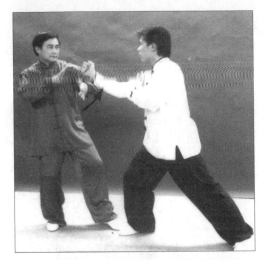 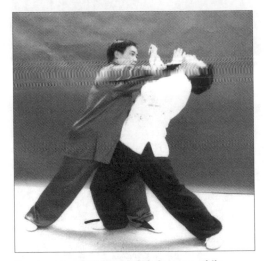

White punches to Gray's head with his right arm. Gray begins lifting his left forearm to intercept.

Gray continues lifting his left forearm while stepping forward with his left foot and striking to White's head with his right palm.

Posture 19: Needle at Sea Bottom (Haidi Zhen)

Movements

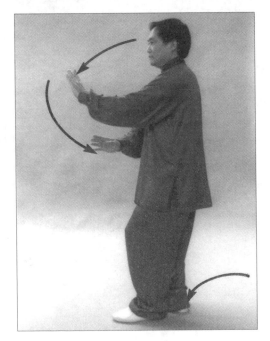

Bring your right foot behind your left and shift all your weight on it, and begin lowering both palms in front of you. (Face west. Inhale.)

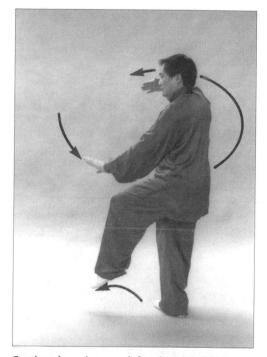

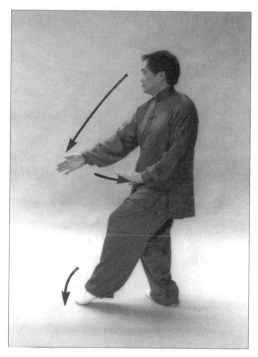

Continue lowering your left palm while lifting your left foot slightly off the floor and circling your right palm back and up until it is next to your ear. (Begin to exhale.)

Pull your left palm next to your waist, touch down on your left foot, and spear down with your right palm. (Face west.)

Key Points

Needle at sea bottom is describing an attack to the opponent's huiyin cavity (sea bottom). The original name is scoop up the needle at sea bottom. The original movements require that your right hand lowers until it reaches the floor. Then scoop up and forward, attacking the opponent's huiyin cavity. In Simplified Taijiquan training, only go as low as you can comfortably. When standing in the empty stance, make sure your right knee is pointing in the same direction as your right foot to prevent unnecessary torsion on your right knee.

Applications

First application

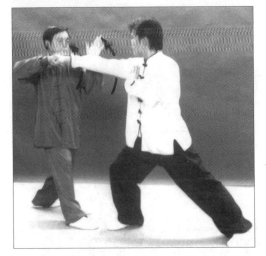 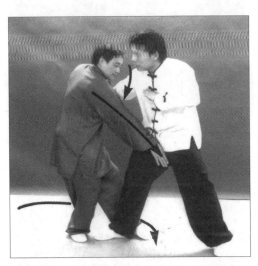

White punches to Gray's chest with his right fist. Gray intercepts with his left forearm.

Gray then pulls White's right arm down with his left palm while stepping his left foot next to White's right foot and spearing his right palm toward White's groin.

Second application

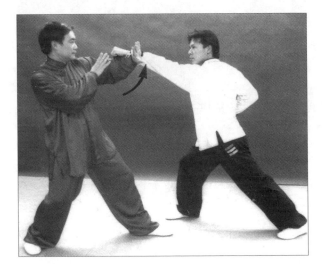

White punches to Gray's head with his left fist. Gray swings his left arm up to intercept.

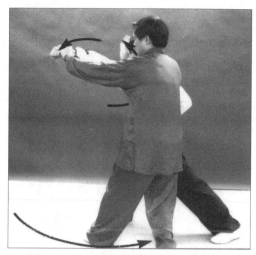

Gray grabs hold of White's left wrist with his left hand and steps forward with his right foot. Gray then turns to his left and locks his right forearm on White's left biceps.

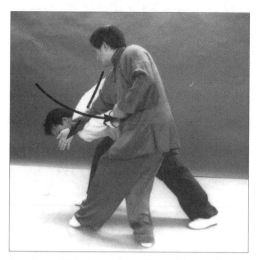

Gray locks White's arm by pulling White's wrist next to his waist and pressing down on White's left biceps with his right forearm.

Third application

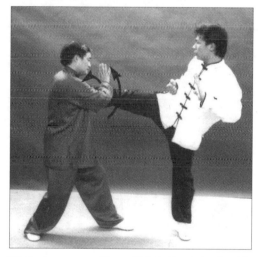

White does a roundhouse kick to Gray's body with his right foot. Gray intercepts White's kick with his right forearm on White's knee while hooking his left arm on White's calf.

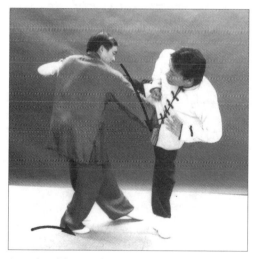

Gray then lifts up White's leg with his left arm while he spears down with his right hand toward White's groin.

Fourth application

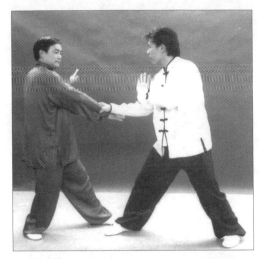

White grabs hold of Gray's right wrist with his right hand.

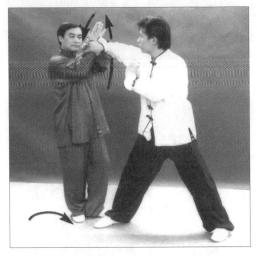

Gray brings his right foot next to his left foot while lifting his right palm to neutralize White's grab. At the same time, Gray grabs hold of White's fingers with his left hand.

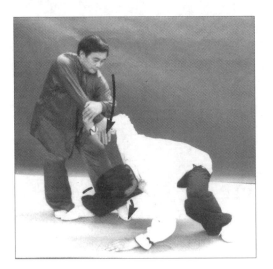

Gray locks White's wrist by extending both hands toward White's body and down.

Posture 20: Fan Through Back (Shan Tong Bei)

Movements

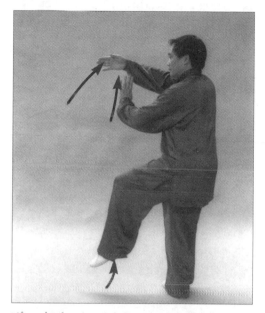

Lift up both palms, left fingers just below your right wrist, while lifting up your left foot slightly. (Inhale.)

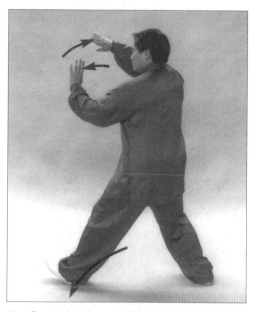

Step forward with your left foot and begin pulling your right palm back and extending your left palm forward. (Begin to exhale.)

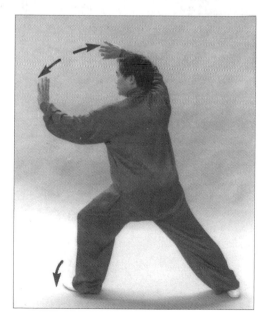

Shift your weight forward into left bow stance, pull your right palm over your head, and extend your left palm in front of you.

Key Points

Shan means fan. The arms are extended, resembling a Chinese fan. *Tong bei* means through the back. It implies that the power is emitted by passing through your back and out to your arms. The traditional Chinese handheld fan is made of leaves similar to palm tree leaves. By cutting the edges of the leaves in a circular pattern, it becomes a handheld fan with the stem as the handle. As power is generated and passed through your back (the stem), it is further manifested by the extended hands (in a circular pattern like the fan).

Applications

First application

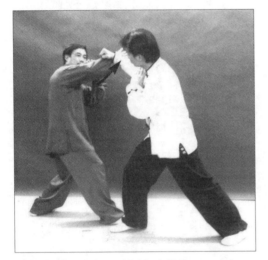 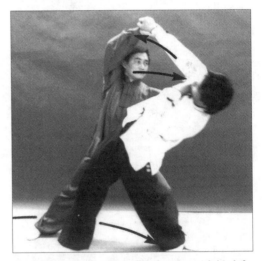

White hook punches with his right fist toward Gray's head. Gray circles his right forearm up to intercept.

Gray then grabs hold of White's wrist with his left hand and pulls it up to his right. At the same time, Gray steps forward with his left foot and strikes White's head with his left palm.

Second application

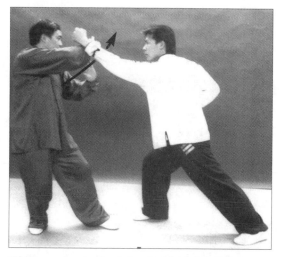

White punches to Gray's head with his left fist. Gray lifts up his right forearm to intercept.

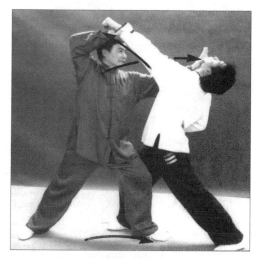

Gray grabs hold of White's left wrist with his right hand and pulls back. At the same time, Gray steps forward with his left foot and strikes White's jaw with his left palm.

SECTION VIII

Posture 21: Turn Body, Deflect, Parry, and Punch (Zhuan Shen Ban Lan Chui)

Movements

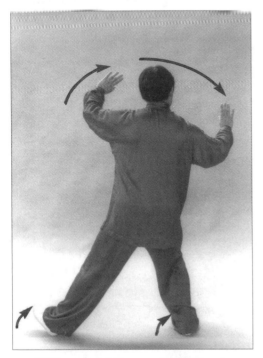

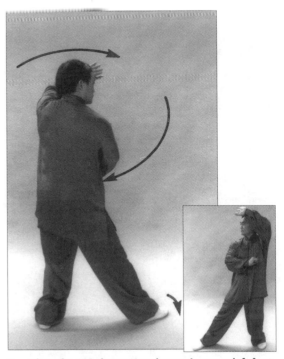

Shift your weight to your right foot and begin making a 180-degree turn to your back. Lift up the ball of your left foot and begin lowering your right palm. (Begin to inhale.)

Complete the 180-degree turn by turning your left foot in and shifting all your weight on it. At the same time, bring your left palm across your head and continue lowering your right palm. Your right palm changes into a fist as it gets next to your body. (See front view.)

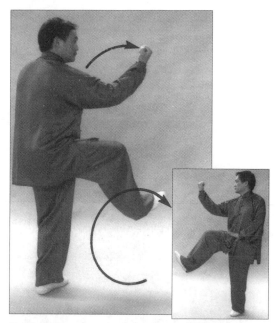

Continue lowering your left palm until it is next to your abdomen while circling your right fist forward and lifting your right foot. (See front view. Face east. Exhale.)

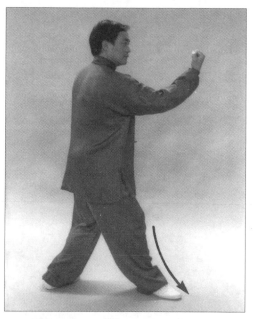

Step down with your right foot, foot turned out. (Begin to inhale.)

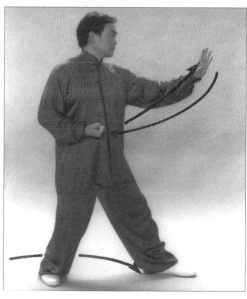

Step forward with your left foot while pulling your right fist to your waist and extending your left palm forward.

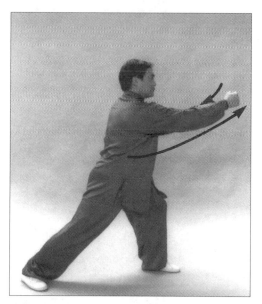

Shift all your weight to your left foot into bow stance while punching with your right fist forward and bringing your left palm next to your right elbow. (Exhale.)

Key Points

This posture is used to defend against an attack from the rear, and then you follow through with an attack. As you circle your right fist in and out, also lift your right foot up and down. Imagine your hand is like the crankshaft on the wheel of a train, rotating the wheel (right foot) in a circular motion.

Applications

First application

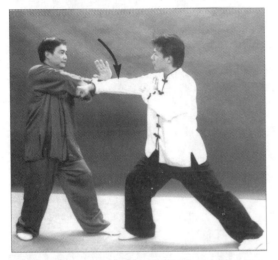

White punches to Gray's chest with his right fist. Gray intercepts by blocking down with his left forearm.

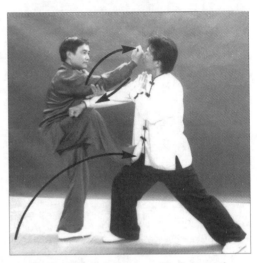

Gray leads White's right arm to his right. At the same time, he strikes with a backfist to White's nose with his right fist and kicks to White's groin with his right foot.

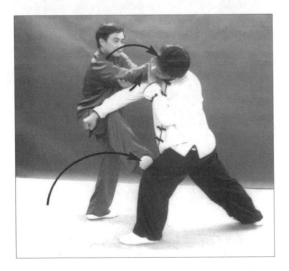

As an alternative, if White had punched with his left foot forward, Gray could kick to White's left knee with his right foot.

Second application

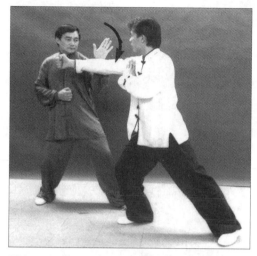

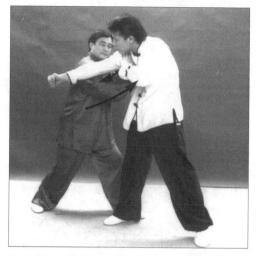

White punches to Gray's chest with his right fist. Gray intercepts with his left forearm.

Gray then steps forward with his left foot and punches to White's chest with his right fist.

Posture 22: Appears Closed (Ru Feng Si Bi)

Movements

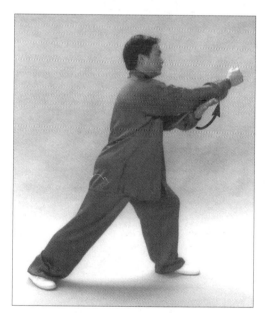

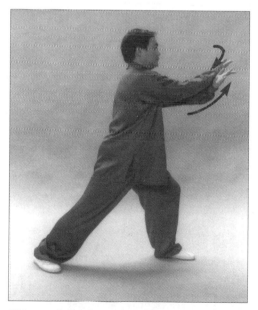

Maintain contact with your left hand and your right elbow, while rotating your left palm to the right side of your right elbow. (Begin to inhale.)

Slide your left palm up your right arm and rotate your right palm until it faces up, both palms open.

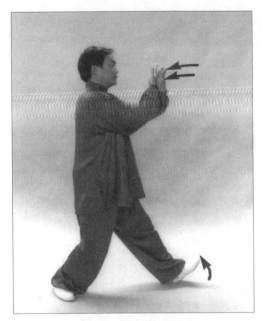

Shift your weight on your right foot, lift up your left foot, and pull both palms closer to your body.

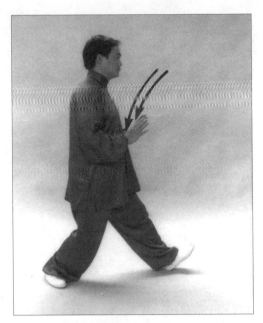

Rotate, separate, and lower your palms until your palms are facing down and next to your abdomen. (Begin to exhale.)

Key Points

Ru feng and *si bi* are two terms with a similar meaning. It implies the sealing motion of the palms down and forward. This posture resembles the push movement in the grasp sparrow's tail posture.

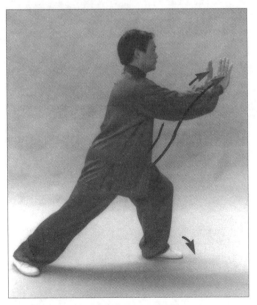

Push forward with both palms while shifting your weight to your left foot into bow stance.

Applications

First application

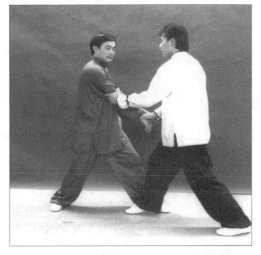

White grabs hold of Gray's right arm with both hands.

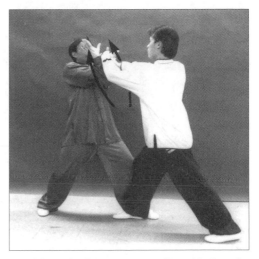

Gray lifts up both arms to neutralize White's grab.

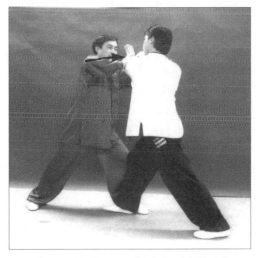

Gray clears White's arm to his left with his left forearm and pushes on White's biceps with his right palm.

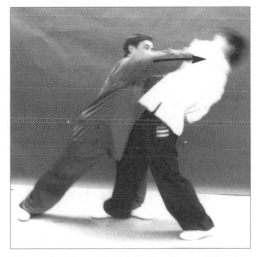

Gray pushes forward with both palms on White's arm and body.

Second application

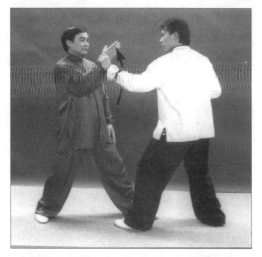

White grabs hold of Gray's right wrist with his left hand.

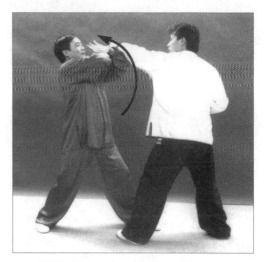

Gray lifts both arms to neutralize White's grab.

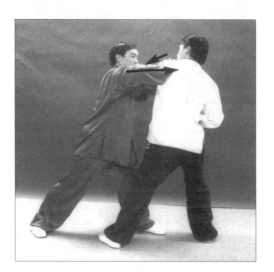

Gray then clears White's left arm to his left while pushing White forward on White's shoulder and chest.

Posture 23: Cross Hands (Shi Zi Shou)

Movements

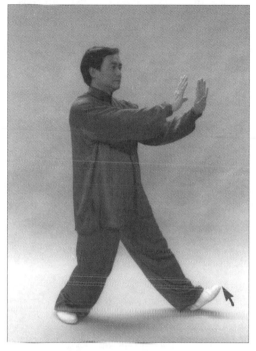

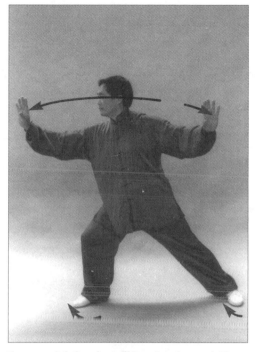

Shift your weight to your right foot, lift up the ball of your left foot, and begin turning your body 180 degrees to your right. (Begin to inhale.)

Turn your left foot in until it points forward. Then turn your right foot out while you rotate and extend your right palm to your right. Pull your left palm to your left slightly.

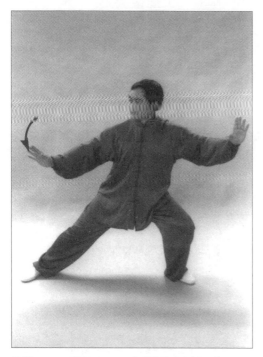

Shift your weight to your left foot and begin lowering your palms. (Begin to exhale.)

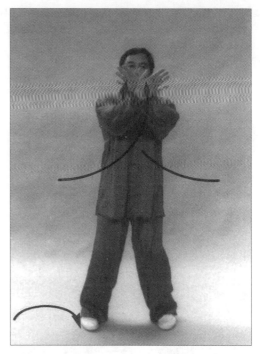

Bring your right foot closer to your left until both feet are shoulder width apart while scooping both palms down and up. Cross wrists in front of your face with the right palm on the outside. Stand up slightly, but keep your knees bent. (Face south.)

Key Points

Shi is the Chinese word for the number ten. The character looks like a cross, and the motion of crossing the arms gives the posture its name.

Applications

First application

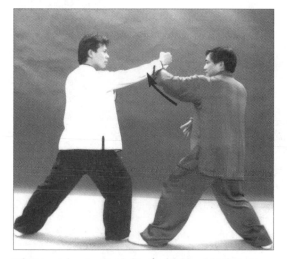

White punches to Gray's head with his right fist. Gray lifts his left arm to intercept.

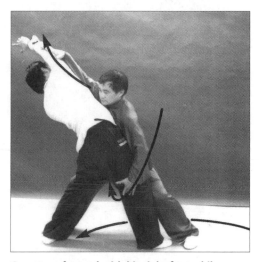

Gray steps forward with his right foot while clearing White's right arm up by extending his right arm forward from under his left arm. At the same time, Gray hooks his left hand behind White's knee.

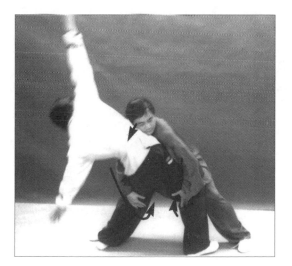

Gray drops White on the floor by sliding his right hand down and hooking on the back of White's left knee. At the same time, Gray presses his head on White's body and pulls both hands back.

Second application

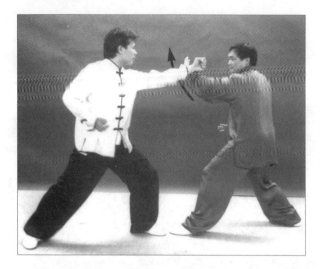

White punches to Gray's head with his left fist. Gray circles his left forearm up to intercept.

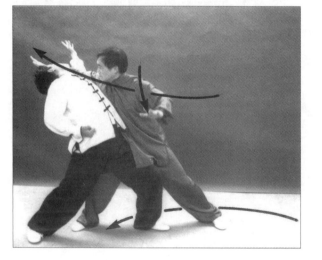

Gray steps forward with his right foot. At the same time, Gray clears White's left arm forward by extending his right arm forward from under his left arm.

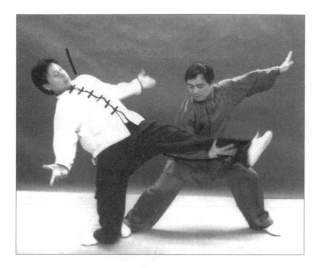

Gray then shifts his weight back to his left leg while hooking his right forearm down under White's left knee and pulls White off balance.

Posture 24: Closing (Shou Shi)

Movements

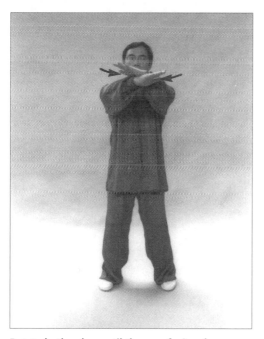

Rotate both palms until they are facing down. (Begin to inhale.)

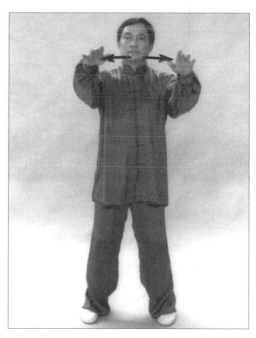

Separate both palms until they are shoulder width apart.

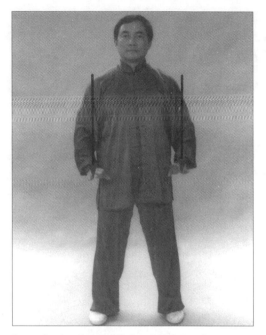

Lower both palms to hip level and stand up completely. (Exhale.)

Bring your left foot next to the right and relax your hands down to your sides.

Key Points

Shou Shi is referring to the ending of the practice. At the end, pause in the posture for a few minutes of standing meditation. Feel the flow of qi in your entire body, letting the qi redistribute, balance, repair, and strengthen your entire body.

CHAPTER FIVE

48 Posture Taijiquan

5.1: **Introduction**

In 1976, another standardized taijiquan (tai chi chuan) sequence was compiled by the Chinese National Athletic Association. The new sequence was called 48 Posture Taijiquan. It broadened the content of the Simplified Taijiquan sequence by adding additional postures from the Yang, Chen, Wu, and Sun styles of Taijiquan. The new postures were modified and performed with the characteristic "flavor" of the Yang Style. Therefore, the same guidelines and principles of Yang Style Taijiquan apply to the 48 Posture Taijiquan. The only exception is that the Simplified Taijiquan sequence is performed at an even pace, and the 48 Posture Taijiquan includes some fast movements. The fast movements are a characteristic of martial arts power emission called *fajin*. These fast transitional movements are placed within * * followed by the phrase *Quick Tempo* placed in parentheses at the end of the description.

5.2: **48 Posture Taijiquan**
48 Posture Taijiquan Posture Names
Commencing (*Qi Shi*)

1. White Crane Spreads Its Wings (*Bai He Liang Chi*)
2. Left Brush Knee and Step Forward (*Zuo Lou Xi Ao Bu*)
3. Left Single Whip (*Zuo Dan Bian*)
4. Left Lute Posture (*Zuo Pipa Shi*)
5. Rollback and Press Posture (*Lu Ji Shi*)
6. Left Deflect, Parry, and Punch (*Zuo Ban Lan Chui*)
7. Left Wardoff, Rollback, Press, and Push (*Zuo Peng Lu Ji An*)
8. Lean on a Diagonal (*Xie Shen Kao*)
9. Fist under Elbow (*Zhou Di Chui*)
10. Reverse Reeling Forearm (*Dao Juan Gong*)

11. Turn Body and Thrust Palm (*Zhuan Shen Tui Zhang*)

12. Right Lute Posture (*You Pipa Shi*)

13. Brush Knee and Punch Down (*Lou Xi Cai Chui*)

14. White Snake Spits Poison (*Bai She Tu Xin*)

15. Slap Foot and Tame the Tiger (*Pai Jiao Fu Hu*)

16. Left Diagonal Backfist (*Zuo Pie Shen Chui*)

17. Piercing Fist and Lower Body (*Chuanquan Xia Shi*)

18. Stand on One Leg and Prop Up Palm (*Du Li Cheng Zhang*)

19. Right Single Whip (*You Dan Bian*)

20. Right Wave Hands Like Clouds (*You Yun Shou*)

21. Left and Right The Wild Horse Parts Its Mane (*Zuo You Fen Zong*)

22. High Pat on Horse (*Gao Tan Ma*)

23. Right Heel Kick (*You Deng Jiao*)

24. Strike to Ears with Both Fists (*Shuang Feng Guan Er*)

25. Left Heel Kick (*Zuo Deng Jiao*)

26. Cover Hand and Strike with Fist (*Yan Shou Liao Quan*)

27. Needle at Sea Bottom (*Haidi Zhen*)

28. Fan through Back (*Shan Tong Bei*)

29. Right and Left Toe Kick (*Zuo You Fen Jiao*)

30. Brush Knee and Step Forward (*Lou Xi Ao Bu*)

31. Step Forward, Grab, and Punch (*Shang Bu Qin Da*)

32. Appears Closed (*Ru Feng Si Bi*)

33. Left Wave Hands Like Clouds (*Zuo Yun Shou*)

34. Right Diagonal Backfist (*You Pie Shen Chui*)

35. Left and Right Shuttle Back and Forth (*Zuo You Chuan Suo*)

36. Step Back and Spear Palm (*Tui Bu Chuan Zhang*)

37. Insubstantial Stance and Press Palm Down (*Xu Bu Ya Zhang*)

38. Stand on One Leg and Lift Palm (*Du Li Tuo Zhang*)

39. Lean in Horse Stance (*Ma Bu Kao*)

40. Turn Body and Large Rollback (*Zhuan Shen Da Lu*)

41. Scoop Palm and Lower Body (*Liao Zhang Xia Shi*)

42. Step Forward and Cross Punch (*Shang Bu Shi Zi Quan*)

43. Stand on One Leg and Ride the Tiger (*Du Li Kua Hu*)

44. Turn Body and Sweep Lotus (*Zhuan Shen Bai Lian*)

45. Pull the Bow and Shoot the Tiger (*Wan Gong She Hu*)

46. Right Deflect, Parry, and Punch (*You Ban Lan Chui*)

47. Right Wardoff, Rollback, Press, and Push (*You Peng Lu Ji An*)

48. Cross Hands (*Shi Zi Shou*)

Closing (*Shou Shi*)

SECTION I

Commencing (Qi Shi)

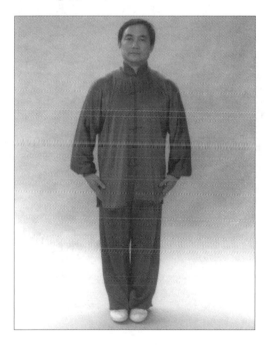

Stand with feet together and hands to your sides. (Face south. Inhale and exhale naturally a few times.)

Key Points

Training the mind is of the highest importance in taijiquan. The preparation posture is to prepare the mind for the physical movements. Before starting the movements, the mind should be calm and steady. Stand naturally upright. Bring your thoughts inward instead of outward. Eyes look evenly forward. Relax your entire body. Imagine there is a waterfall gently pouring over your head. As the water passes through your body, tension is released in your head, neck, shoulders, chest, spine, elbows, hands, hips, knees, ankles, feet, and toes, and then into the ground. Repeat this process until you feel completely relaxed and calm.

Before starting the postures, touch your tongue to the roof of your mouth. As saliva is being generated, swallow it and use your mind to follow the saliva down your throat to your stomach. Then bring your attention to your dan tian, your body's center of gravity.

Movements

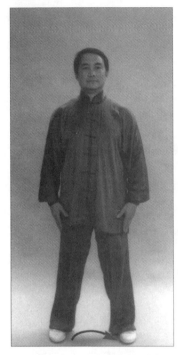 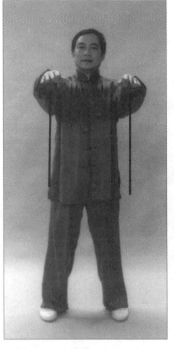 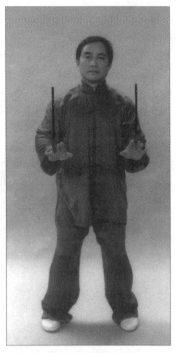

Bend your knees slightly, and then step to your left with your left leg, shoulder width apart. (Begin to inhale.)

Rotate your palms as you raise up your arms slowly to shoulder level, palms facing down.

Pull your arms in slightly and lower them to abdomen level as you bend your knees slightly. (Exhale.)

Posture 1: White Crane Spreads Its Wings (Bai He Liang Chi)

Movements

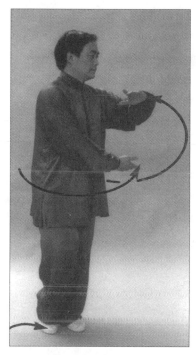 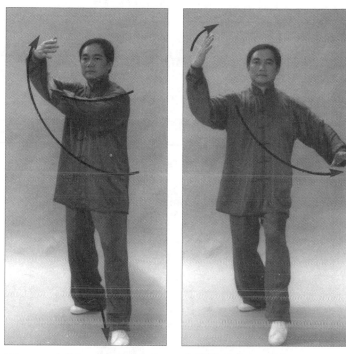

Bring your right foot next to your left while your left palm circles clockwise up, palm down. At the same time, turn your body slightly to your left and rotate your right palm up.

Bring your left foot a half step forward. Shift all your weight onto your right foot. At the same time, bring your right palm up past your left elbow and lift your left foot up slightly. Complete the movement by lowering your left palm down to waist level, palm down. Raise your right palm up to head level, palm facing inward, and touch down with your left foot into empty stance.

Posture 2: Left Brush Knee and Step Forward (Zuo Lou Xi Ao Bu)
Movements

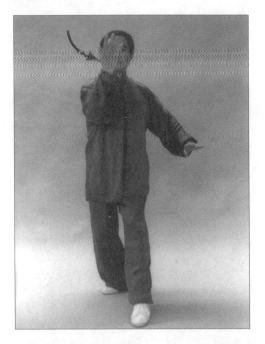

Turn your body slightly to your left while rotating your right palm to face you.

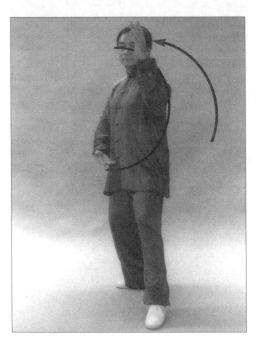

Turn your body to your right while lowering your right hand down to your waist and circling your left arm up with your palm facing to your right.

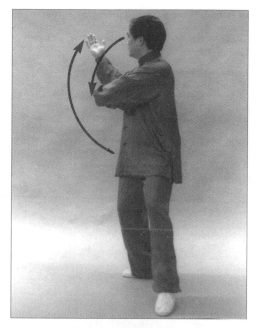

Turn your body farther to your right while lowering your left hand and circling your right hand up. Eyes look at your right palm.

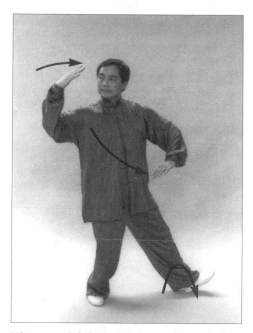

Lift up your left foot slightly, step forward while beginning to brush your left palm across your left knee, and extend your right palm forward.

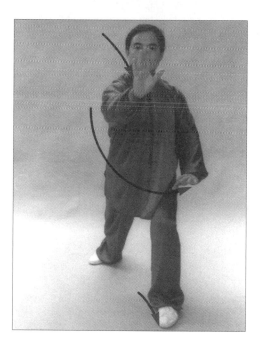

Shift your weight to your left foot into bow stance and extend your right palm forward.

Posture 3: Left Single Whip (Zuo Dan Bian)

Movements

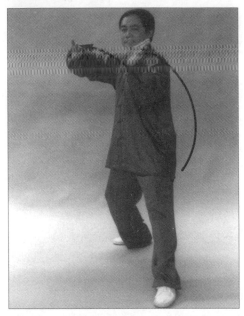

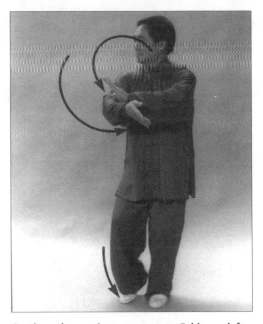

Shift your weight back to your right leg while rotating your right palm to face right and pull back. At the same time, lift your left palm up to shoulder level.

Continue the previous movements. Fold your left forearm in next to your chest while making a big clockwise circle with your right palm until it is under your left palm. As you move your arms, shift all your weight to your left leg and bring the ball of your right foot next to your left.

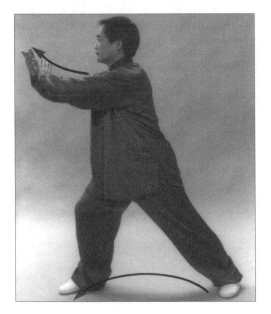

Step to your right with your right foot into bow stance while extending both arms forward. (Step west.)

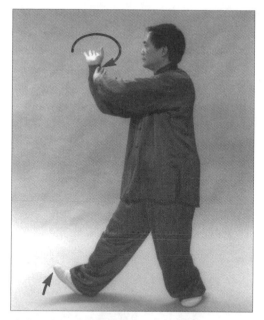

Shift your weight back to your left leg and lift up your right foot. At the same time, begin rotating your right forearm to your right by pivoting on your elbow with your palm facing up.

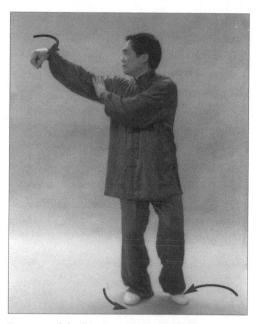

Turn your right foot in until it is facing forward, shift your weight on it, and bring your left foot next to your right. At the same time, continue the rotation of your right forearm by bringing your palm up to head level. Then extend it to your right and form a hook.

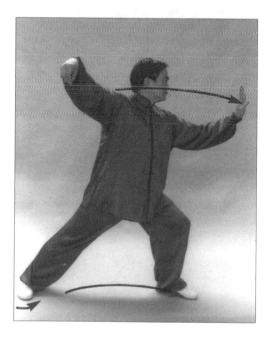

Complete the single whip posture by stepping to your left, the same as the single whip, posture 11, in the Simplified Taijiquan sequence. (Step east.)

Posture 4: Left Lute Posture (Zuo Pipa Shi)

Movements

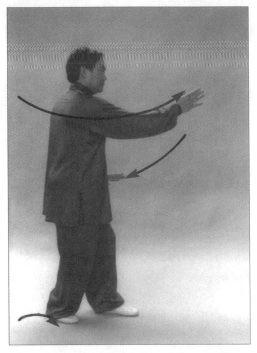

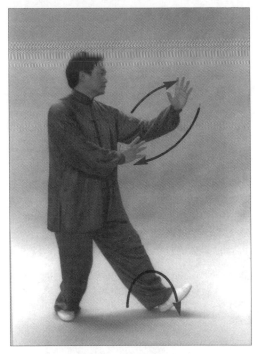

Bring your right foot behind your left and shift your weight on it while swinging your right hand forward and lowering your left palm to your side.

Lift up your left foot and touch down with your heel while circling your right palm down and circling your left palm forward. Both palms face inward.

Posture 5: Rollback and Press Posture (Lu Ji Shi)

Movements

Rollback, left side

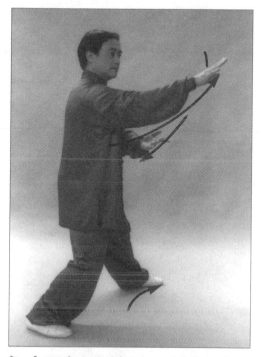

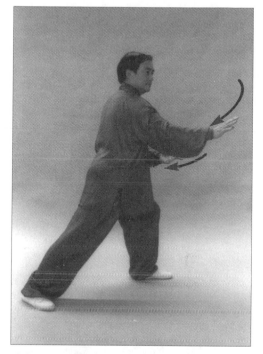

Step forward to your left corner while extending and circling your right palm to your right, over your left palm. At the same time, turn your left palm up and bring it closer to your body. Both palms move in a clockwise arc. (Step northeast.)

Shift your weight to your left leg while lowering both palms in the direction of your left knee.

Press, right side

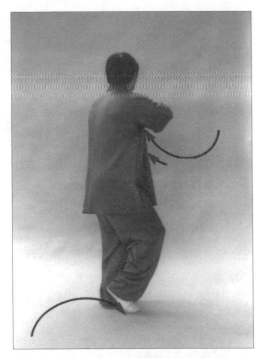 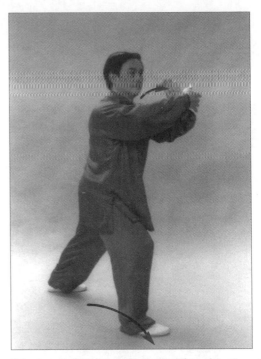

Shift all your weight to your left leg and bring the ball of your right foot next to it. At the same time, raise both palms up: your right palm next to your chest with fingers pointing to your left and your left palm facing your head with fingers pointing up.

Bring your left palm next to your right wrist, step to your front right corner with your right foot, and extend both palms forward. (Step southeast.)

Rollback, right side

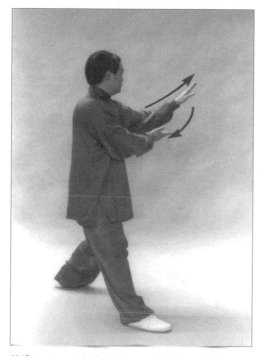

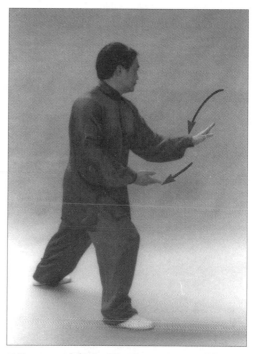

Shift your weight back to your left leg while circling both palms counterclockwise.

Shift your weight back to your right leg while lowering both palms in the direction of your right knee.

Press, left side

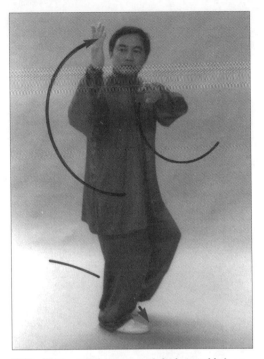 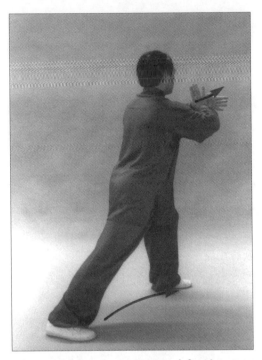

Shift all your weight to your right leg and bring your left foot next to it. At the same time, raise both palms up: your left palm next to your chest with fingers pointing to your right and your right palm facing your head with fingers pointing up.

Bring your right palm next to your left wrist, step to your front left corner with your left foot, and extend both palms forward. (Step northeast.)

Rollback, left side

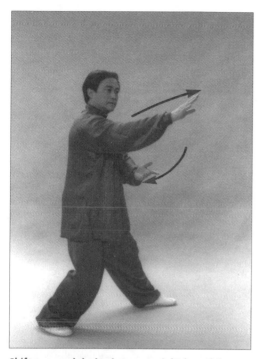

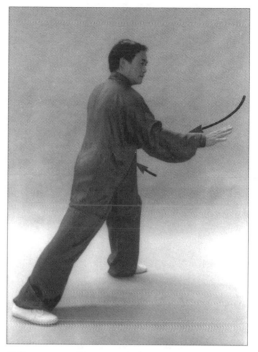

Shift your weight back to your right leg while extending and circling your right palm to your right, over your left palm. At the same time, turn your left palm up and bring it closer to your body. Both palms move in a clockwise arc. (Step northeast.)

Shift your weight to your left leg while lowering both palms in the direction of your left knee.

Press, right side

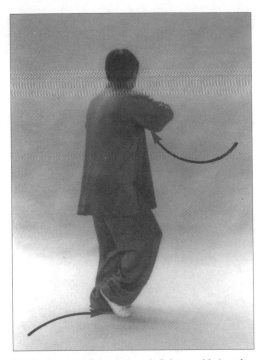

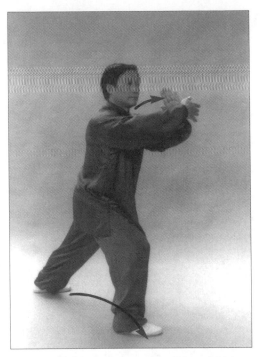

Shift all your weight to your left leg and bring the ball of your right foot next to it. At the same time, raise both palms up: your right palm next to your chest with fingers pointing to your left and your left palm facing your head with fingers pointing up.

Bring your left palm next to your right wrist, step to your front right corner with your right foot, and extend both palms forward. (Step southeast.)

Posture 6: Left Deflect, Parry, and Punch (Zuo Ban Lan Chui)

Movements

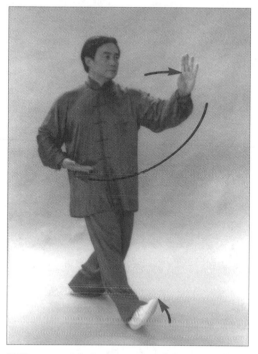

Shift your weight back to your left leg, extend your left palm forward, and pull your right palm back next to your waist.

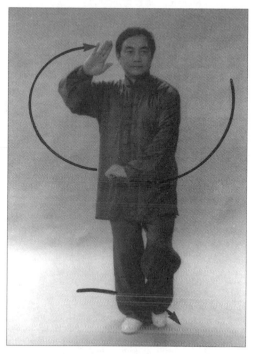

Turn your right foot out, shift all your weight on it, and touch the ball of your left foot next to it. At the same time, hold your left hand in a fist and lower it to your waist level. Then circle your right palm back and up to head level.

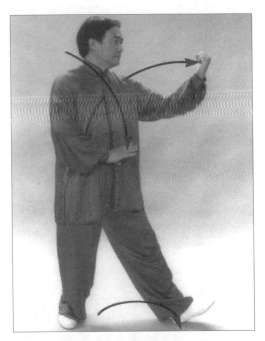

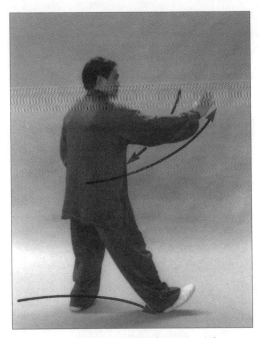

Continue the previous arm movements. Lower your right palm next to your waist while circling your left fist up and forward. At the same time, lift up your left foot slightly and place it down in front of you with your heel touching the floor. (Step east.)

Turn your left foot out and shift your weight on it. Then step forward with your right leg while pulling your left fist back to your waist and extending your right palm forward.

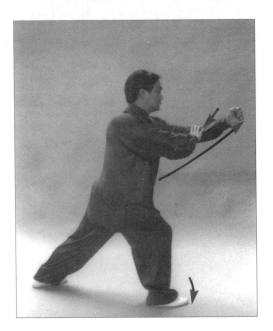

Shift your weight to your right leg while punching forward with your left fist.

Posture 7: Left Wardoff, Rollback, Press, and Push (Zuo Peng Lu Ji An)

Movements

Wardoff, left side

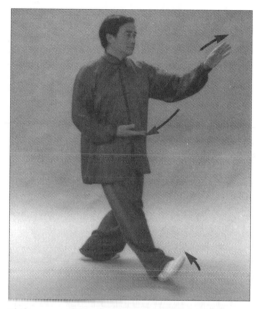

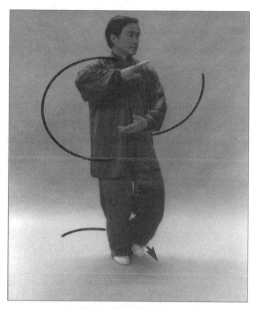

Shift your weight back to your left leg. At the same time, pull your right palm back next to your waist and open your left palm.

Turn your right foot out, shift your weight to your right leg, and bring your left foot next to it. At the same time, circle your right palm counterclockwise up until it is in front of your chest, palm down, and bring your left palm next to your waist, palm up.

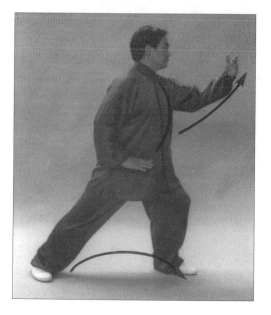

Shift your weight forward into a left bow stance and complete the previous arm movements.

Rollback, left side

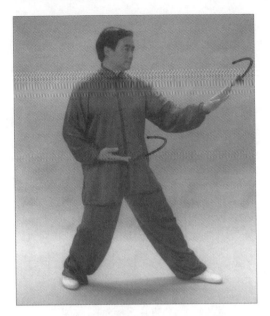

Rotate both palms clockwise, and then shift your weight back to your right foot. This is the left rollback posture.

Press, left side

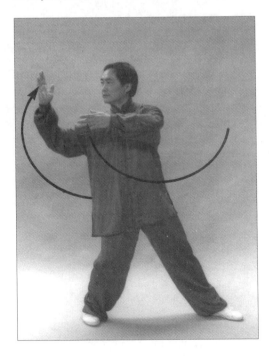

Lower both palms down and up to the back.

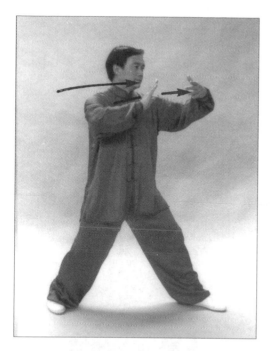

Continue the circular movements of your arms and begin extending them forward.

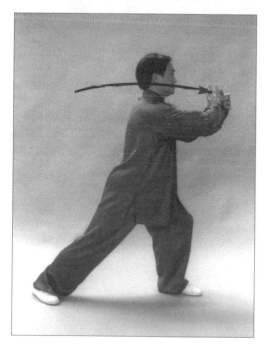

Touch your right palm to your left wrist, and extend both palms forward while shifting your weight to your left foot. This is the completion of the left press posture.

Push, left side

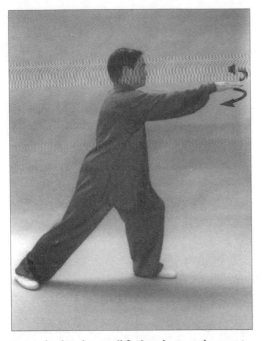

Rotate both palms until facing down and separate them while shifting your weight to your right foot.

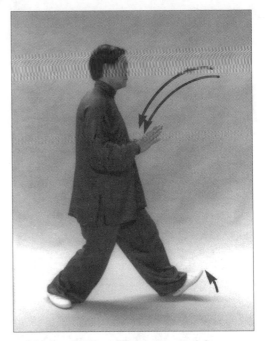

Pull both palms in and down to your abdomen.

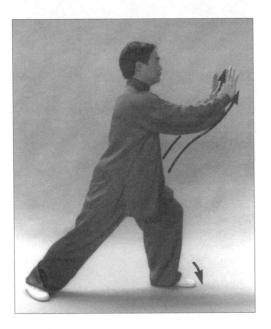

Push forward with both palms while shifting your weight to your left foot. This is the completion of the left push posture.

SECTION II

Posture 8: Lean on a Diagonal (Xie Shen Kao)

Movements

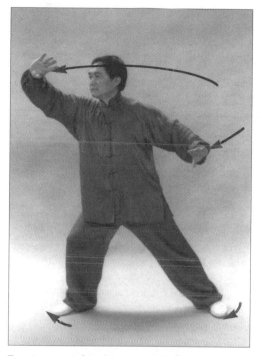

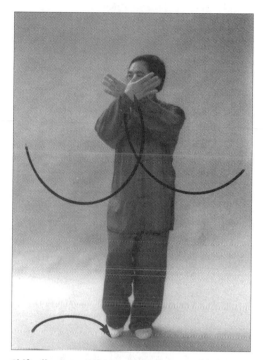

Turn to your right, pivot your right foot out, and shift your weight on it while extending your right arm to your right.

Shift all your weight on your left leg and bring your right foot next to your left. At the same time, lower both palms, and then raise and cross them in front of your chest, right palm on the outside.

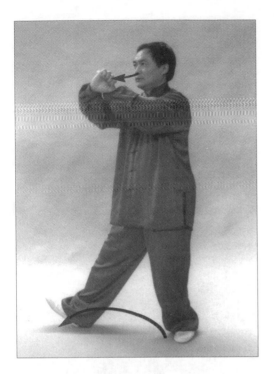

Step to your front right corner with your right foot while holding both hands in, fists facing out. (Step northwest.)

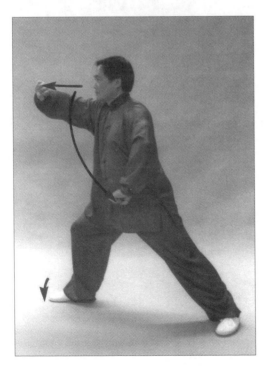

Shift your weight to your right leg into a bow stance while extending your right forearm forward and lowering your left fist next to waist level.

Posture 9: Fist Under Elbow (Zhou Di Chui)

Movements

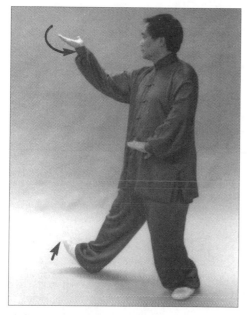

Shift your weight back to your left leg, drop your right elbow, open your right palm, and rotate your right palm up. At the same time, open your left palm.

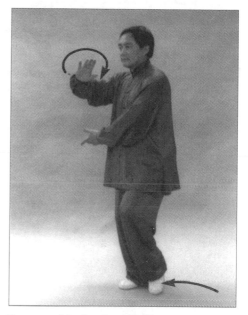

Turn your right foot in, shift all your weight on it, and bring your left foot next to your right. At the same time, bring both palms next to your chest as if you were holding a ball.

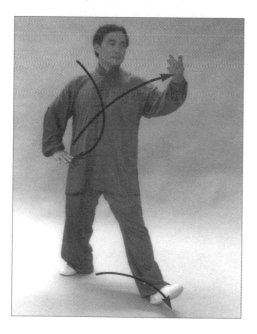

Step to your left with your left foot, and extend your left forearm up and forward. At the same time, lower your right palm next to your waist. (Step southeast.)

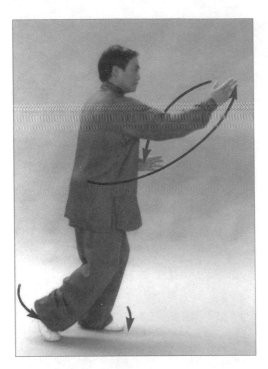

Turn your left foot out, shift all your weight on it, and bring your right foot behind your left foot. At the same time, extend your right palm up and forward, and lower your left palm to your waist.

Shift all your weight to your right leg. Lift up your left foot and touch down on your heel. At the same time, extend your left palm forward as your right hand becomes a fist and lowers until it is under your left elbow. (Face east.)

Posture 10: Reverse Reeling Forearm (Dao Juan Gong)

Also Called Repulse Monkey (Dao Nian Hou)

Movements

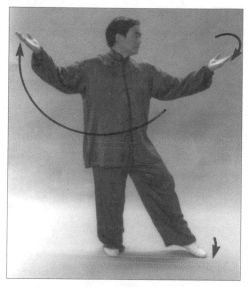

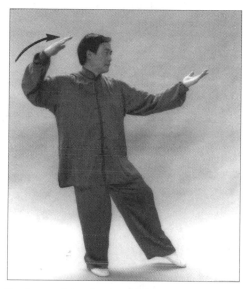

From the previous movement, open your right hand. Circle it back, lift it, and extend it behind you while rotating both palms up. Touch down with your left foot.

Bend your right elbow and begin stepping back with your left foot.

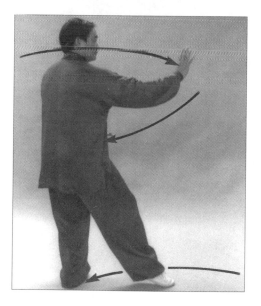

Complete stepping with your left foot behind your right one. Pivot on the balls of your feet and turn your body toward your left while pulling your left palm next to your waist and extending your right palm forward.

Reverse Reeling Forearm, left side

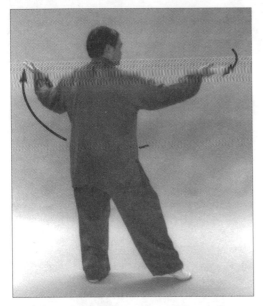

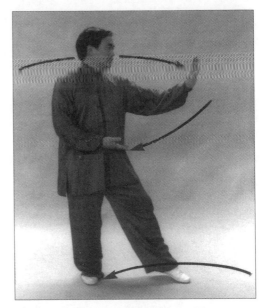

Extend your left arm out and up while rotating both palms up.

Bend your left elbow and step back with your right foot behind your left one. Pivot on the balls of your feet and turn your body toward your right while pulling your right palm next to your waist and extending your left palm forward.

Reverse Reeling Forearm, right side

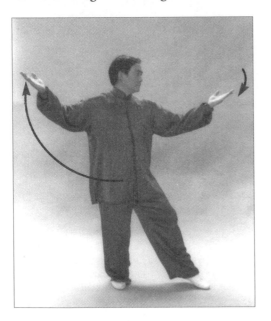

Extend your right arm out and up while rotating both palms up.

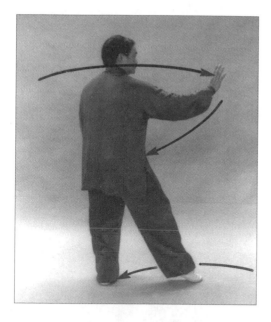

Bend your right elbow and step back with your left foot behind your right one. Pivot on the balls of your feet and turn your body toward your left while pulling your left palm next to your waist and extending your right palm forward.

Reverse Reeling Forearm, left side

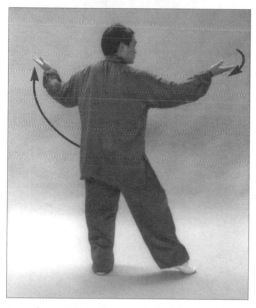

Extend your left arm out and up while rotating both palms up.

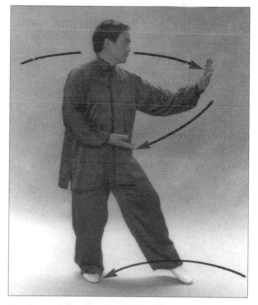

Bend your left elbow and step back with your right foot behind your left one. Pivot on the balls of your feet and turn your body toward your right while pulling your right palm next to your waist and extending your left palm forward.

Posture 11: Turn Body and Thrust Palm (Zhuan Shen Tui Zhang)

Movements

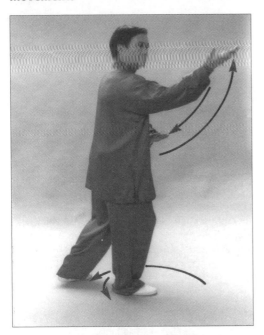

Step back with your left foot. At the same time, lower your left palm next to your body and lift up your right palm to head level.

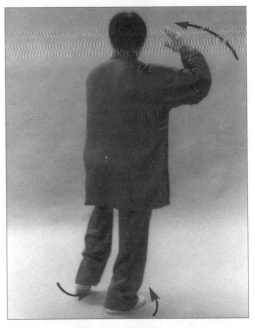

Turn 135 degrees to your left by pivoting on the heel of your right foot and the ball of your left foot. At the same time, bend your elbow and bring your right palm next to your right ear.

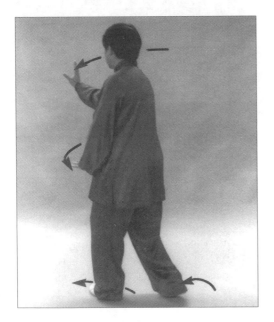

Take a small step forward with your left foot and shift most of your weight on it. Right foot follows up with a small step, touching down on the ball of your foot. At the same time, thrust your right palm forward and bring your left palm next to your waist. (Step northwest.)

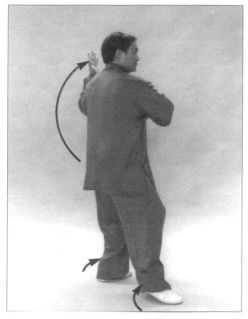

Turn to your back by pivoting on the ball of your right foot and the heel of your left foot. At the same time, bring your right palm next to your body and lift up your left palm to eye level with your elbow bent.

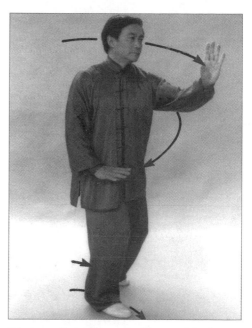

Take a small step forward with your right foot and shift most of your weight on it. Left foot follows up with a small step, touching down on the ball of your foot. At the same time, thrust your left palm forward and bring your right palm next to your waist. (Step southeast.)

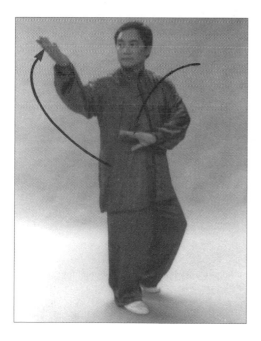

Bring your left palm next to your body and lift up your right palm to your eye level with your elbow bent.

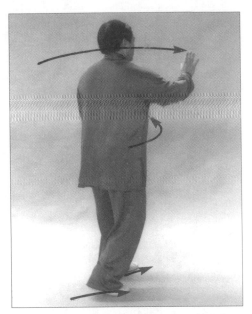

Take a small step to your left with your left foot and shift most of your weight on it. Right foot follows up with a small step, touching down on the ball of your foot. At the same time, thrust your right palm forward and bring your left palm next to your waist. (Step northeast.)

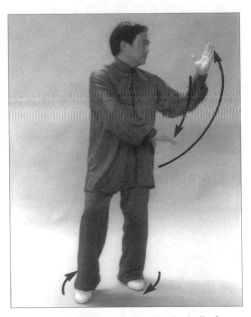

Turn to your back by pivoting on the ball of your right foot and the heel of your left foot. At the same time, bring your right palm next to your body and lift up your left palm to eye level with your elbow bent.

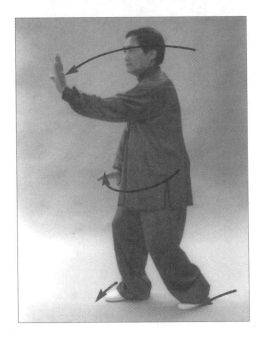

Take a small step forward with your right leg and shift most of your weight on it. Left foot follows up with a small step, touching down on the ball of your foot. At the same time, thrust your left palm forward and bring your right palm next to your waist. (Step southwest.)

Posture 12: Right Lute Posture (You Pipa Shi)

Movements

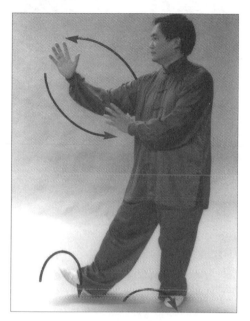

Step back to your back left corner with your left foot and shift your weight on it as you lift up your right foot and touch down on your heel. At the same time, pull your left palm back and extend your right palm forward. (Face west.)

Posture 13: Brush Knee and Punch Down (Lou Xi Cai Chui)

Movements

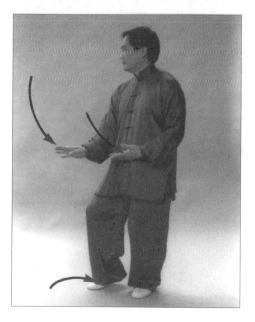

Rotate your right palm until it faces down and rotate your left palm until it faces up. Then lower both palms down to your waist. At the same time, bring your right foot closer to your left with the ball of your right foot touching the floor.

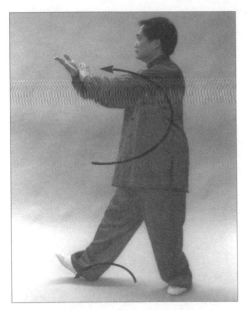

Bring both palms up to shoulder level with your left palm touching the inside of your right wrist. Then extend both palms forward while stepping forward with your right foot.

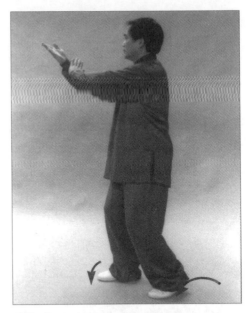

Shift all your weight to your right foot and bring your left foot closer to your right foot.

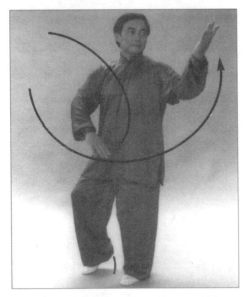

Shift all your weight to your left leg and lift your right heel off the floor. At the same time, lower your left palm down and then up to head level, and bend your right elbow, lowering your right palm down next to your waist.

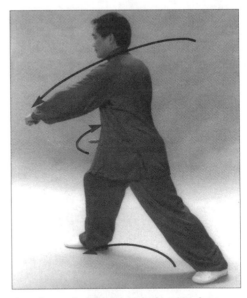

Step forward with your right foot into bow stance. At the same time, punch down with a left fist and pull your right palm next to your waist.

SECTION III

Posture 14: White Snake Spits Poison (Bai She Tu Xin)

Movements

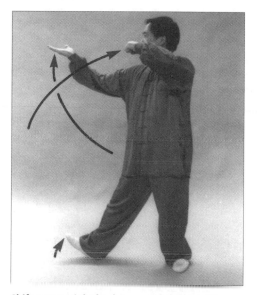

Shift your weight back to your left leg while lifting up your right palm and left fist to head level.

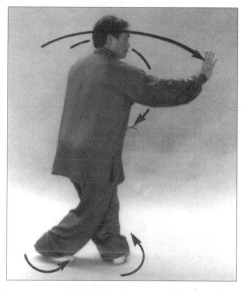

Turn to your back by turning your right foot in, then lifting and turning your left foot out. At the same time, pull your left palm next to your waist, palm down, and extend your right palm forward. (Face east.)

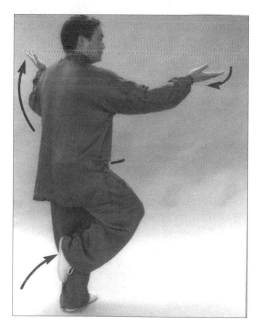

Lift up your right foot while extending your left palm up and turning your right palm up.

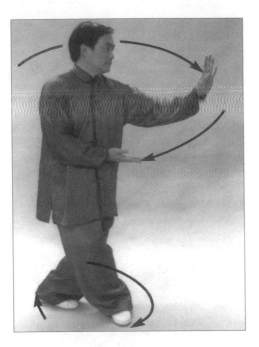

Step down with your right foot and turn your foot out. At the same time, pull your right palm next to your waist and extend your left palm forward.

Posture 15: Slap Foot and Tame the Tiger (Pai Jiao Fu Hu)

Movements

Slap Foot and Tame the Tiger, left side

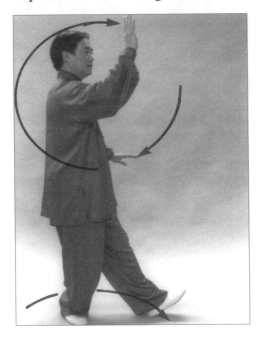

Step forward with your left foot while circling your right palm down and back up to head level.

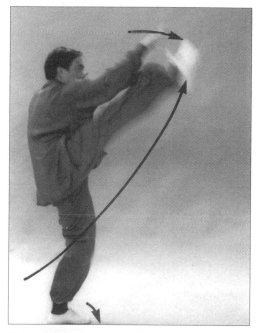

Shift your weight to your left leg. *Then kick your right foot up and slap it with your right palm.* (*Quick Tempo*)

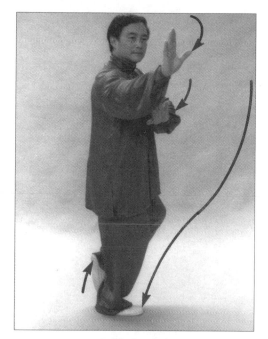

Bring your right foot down next to your left and shift all your weight on it. The left foot touches the floor lightly. At the same time, rotate both palms clockwise to your right. (*Quick Tempo*)

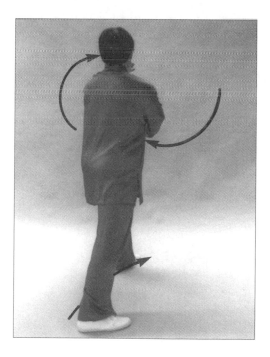

Step to your left with your left foot into bow stance. At the same time, lower both hands in fists over your knee. Continue the movement of your left fist up to head level and bring your right fist next to your chest. (Step north.)

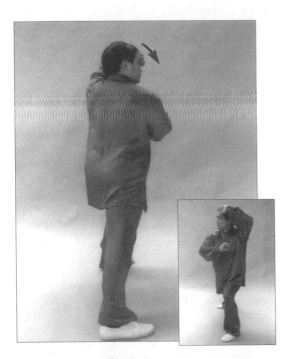

Bend both elbows, pull both fists closer to your body, and turn your head to your right. (See front view.)

Slap Foot and Tame the Tiger, right side

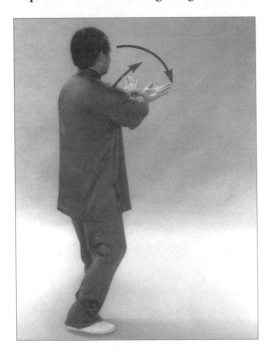

Shift your weight back to your right leg while lowering your left arm and extending your right palm over your left.

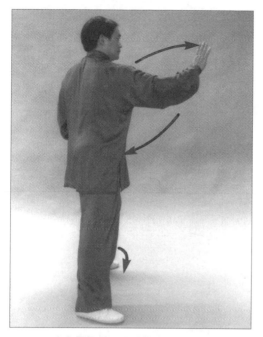

Turn your left foot in and shift your weight forward to your left leg while extending your right palm in an arc to your right. At the same time, bring your left palm down next to your waist, palm up.

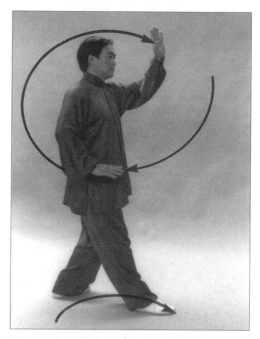

Bring your right foot next to your left foot as you step to your right. At the same time, lower your right palm next to your waist and circle your left palm back and up until it is in front of you. (Step east.)

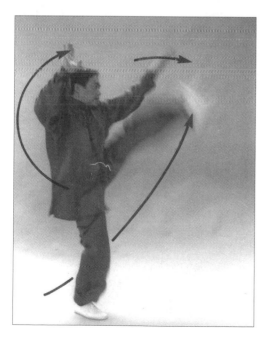

Shift all your weight to your right leg. Then *kick up with your left foot, and slap it with your left palm while circling your right palm back and up.* (*Quick Tempo*)

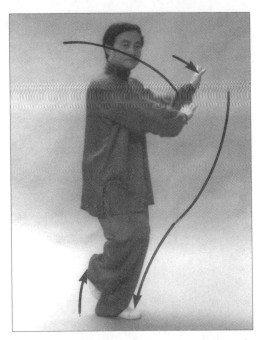

Bring your left foot down next to your right and shift all your weight on it. Right foot touches the floor lightly. At the same time, rotate both palms counterclockwise to your left. (* *Quick Tempo*)

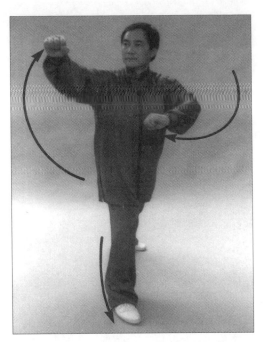

Step to your right with your right foot into bow stance. At the same time, lower both hands in fists over your knee. Continue the movement of your right fist up to head level and bring your left fist next to your chest. (Step south.)

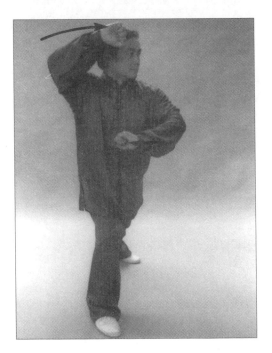

Bend both elbows, pulling both fists closer to your body, and turn your head to your left.

Posture 16: Left Diagonal Back Fist (Zuo Pie Shen Chui)

Movements

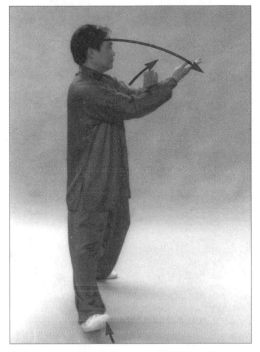 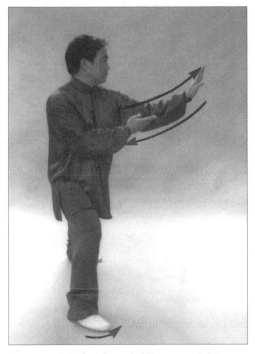

Shift your weight back to your left leg while lowering your right arm. At the same time, open both fists and begin extending your left palm over your right one.

Turn your right foot in and shift your weight forward. At the same time, pull your right palm back next to your chest and extend your left palm forward.

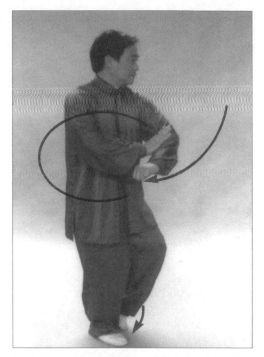 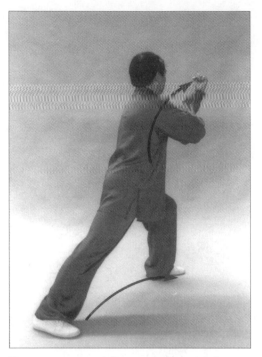

Shift all your weight to your right leg and touch the ball of your left foot next to your right. At the same time, lower both arms and place your right palm on top of your left forearm. The left hand is in a fist.

Step to your upper left corner with your left foot. At the same time, circle your left fist up and forward in front of you. (Step northeast.)

Posture 17: Piercing Fist and Lower Body (Chuanquan Xia Shi)

Movements

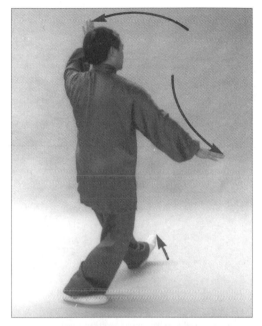

Shift your weight back to your right leg while circling your left palm counterclockwise to your left and circling your right palm counterclockwise to your right.

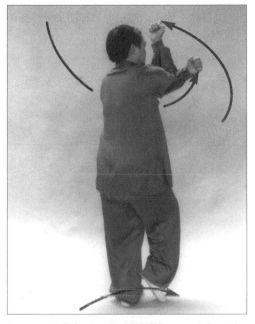

Turn your left foot out and shift your weight on it while touching the ball of your right foot next to your left foot. At the same time, continue circling your right arm up and left arm down. Both hands are held in fists, with your right elbow between your body and your left forearm.

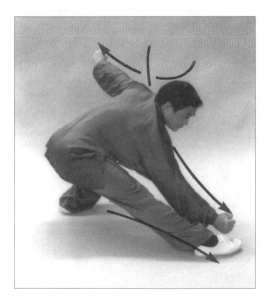

Step to your upper right corner with your right foot and lower your body. At the same time, extend your left fist to your left and extend your right fist down along the inside of your right leg until it is next to your right foot. (Step southeast.)

Posture 18: Stand on One Leg and Prop Up Palm (Du Li Cheng Zhang)

Movements

Stand on One Leg and Prop Up Palm, left side

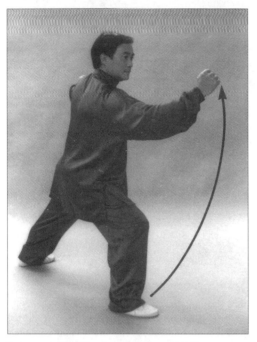 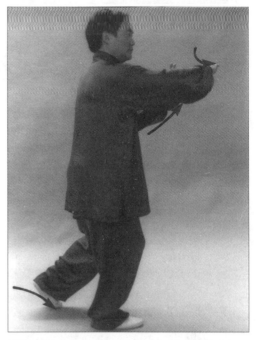

Turn your right foot out slightly and shift your weight forward into bow stance. At the same time, lift up your right fist.

Shift all your weight to your right leg and begin lifting up your left knee. At the same time, bend your right elbow in and bring your left palm between your body and your right arm. Right palm faces down and left palm faces in.

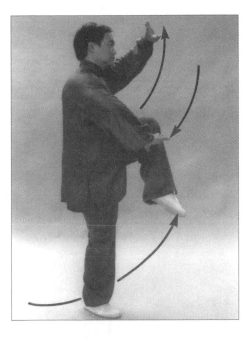

Lift up your left knee while extending your left palm up and right palm down. (Face east.)

Stand on One Leg and Prop Up Palm, right side

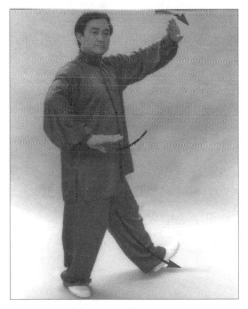

Step down with your left foot.

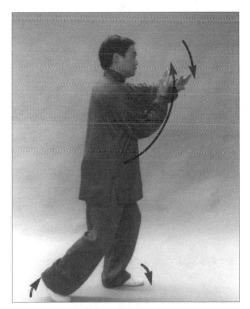

Shift all your weight to your left leg and begin lifting up your right knee. At the same time, lower your right forearm, bringing your right palm between your body and your left arm. The left palm faces down and the right palm faces in.

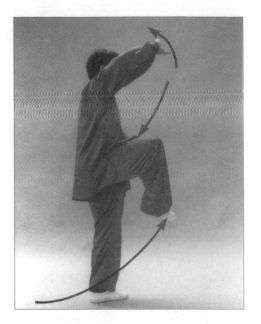

Lift up your right knee while extending your right palm up and left palm down.

Posture 19: Right Single Whip (You Dan Bian)

Movements

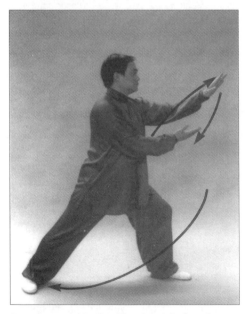

Step down and back with your right foot into bow stance. At the same time, extend your left palm forward and lower your right palm. Right palm faces up and left palm faces down.

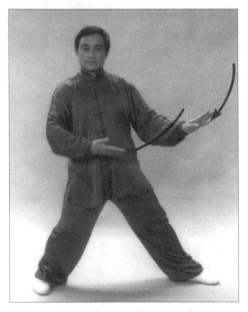

Shift your weight back and lower both palms.

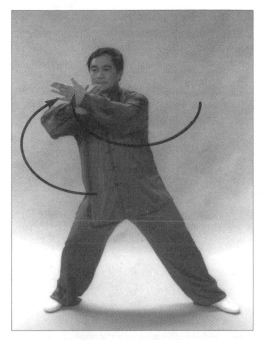

Circle both palms up to head level with your right palm touching the inside of your left wrist.

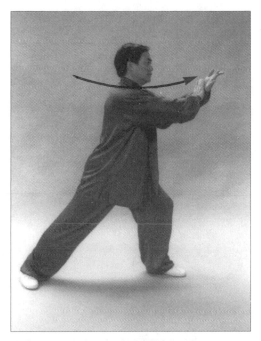

Shift your weight to your left leg into bow stance while circling and extending both palms forward.

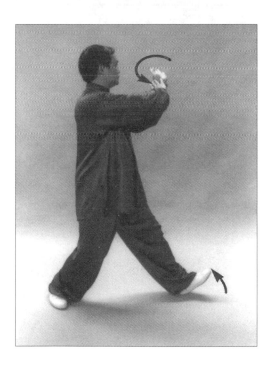

Shift your weight back to your right leg and lift up the ball of your left foot. At the same time, begin making a complete horizontal circle to your left with your left palm facing up.

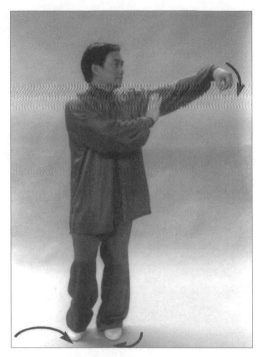

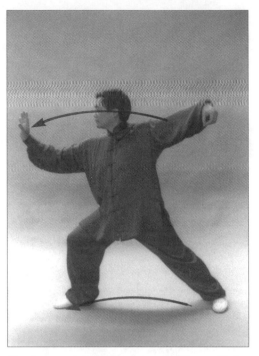

Turn your left foot in, shift your weight on it, and touch the ball of your right foot next to your left. As you complete the palm circle, extend your left arm to your left side and hook your hand down. Place your right palm next to your armpit.

Step to your right. Shift your weight forward into bow stance while rotating and extending your right palm in front of you. (Step west.)

SECTION IV

Posture 20: Right Wave Hands Like Clouds (You Yun Shou)
Movements

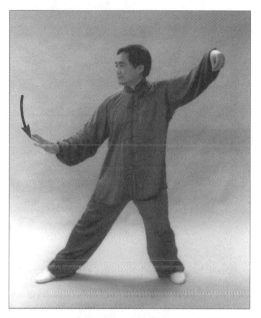

Lower your right hand and shift your weight to your left leg.

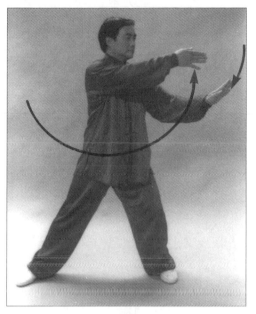

Turn your right foot in until it points forward while beginning to circle your right palm up. Open your left palm and begin lowering it.

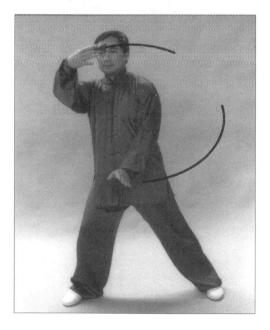

Continue circling your right palm up and across your face while lowering your left palm.

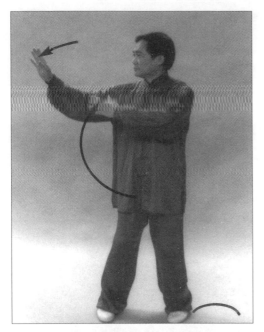

Continue with the previous palm movements—extending your right palm to your right and lifting your left palm—while you bring your left foot closer to your right foot.

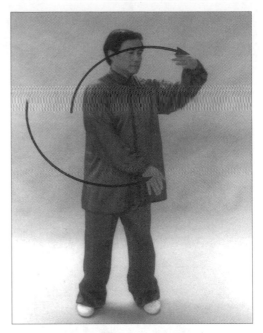

Turn your upper body to your left while continuing to circle your left palm up and across your face and lowering your right palm.

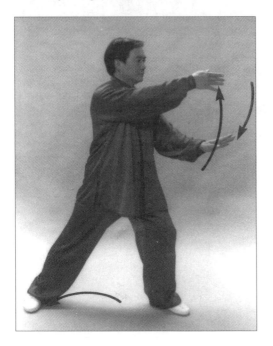

Step to your right with your right foot while circling your right palm up and begin lowering your left palm.

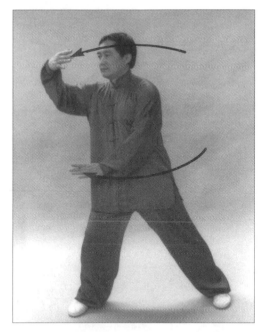

Continue circling your right palm up and across your face while lowering your left palm.

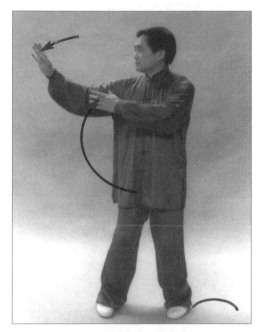

Continue with the previous palm movements—extending your right palm to your right and lifting your left palm—while you bring your left foot closer to your right foot.

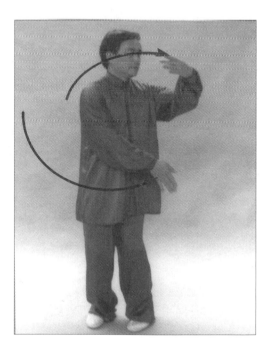

Turn your upper body to your left while continuing to circle your left palm up and across your face and lowering your right palm.

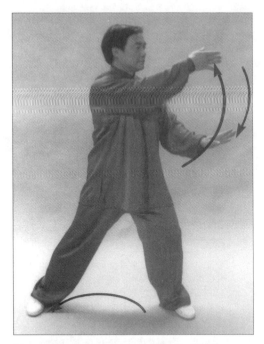

Step to your right with your right foot while circling your right palm up and begin lowering your left palm.

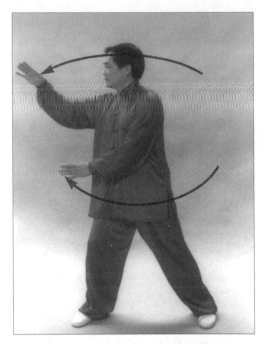

Continue circling your right palm up and across your face while lowering your left palm.

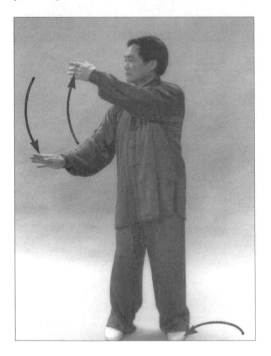

Continue with the previous palm movements—extending your right palm to your right and lifting your left palm—while you bring your left foot closer to your right foot.

Posture 21: Left and Right, The Wild Horse Parts Its Mane (Zuo You Fen Zong)

Movements

The Wild Horse Parts Its Mane, right side

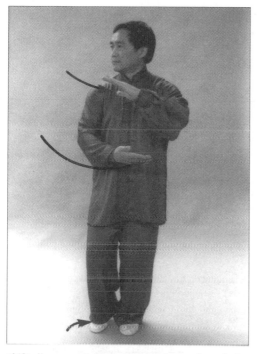 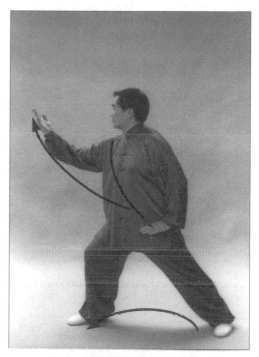

Shift all your weight to your left leg and touch the ball of your right foot next to your left one. At the same time, bring both palms next to your body with palms facing each other.

Step forward with your right foot, touching down with your heel first. Begin turning your body to your right while pulling your left hand down and extending your right hand forward. Shift your weight forward into a right bow stance while extending your right palm forward until it is at eye level and lowering your left palm until it is next to your hip.

The Wild Horse Parts Its Mane, left side

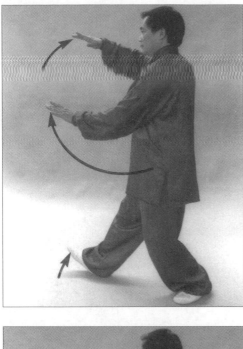

Shift your weight back to your left foot. Lift up the ball of your right foot. Turn your right foot out and shift your weight on it while you begin to turn your body to your right. Rotate your right palm until it is facing down and let your left hand circle forward with the rotation of your body. Look in the direction of your right hand.

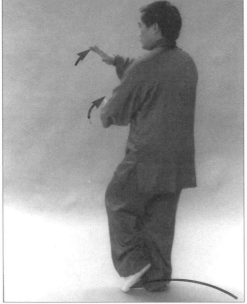

Bring your left foot forward, next to your right one, while bringing your right palm next to your chest, palm down, and bringing your left palm next to your abdomen, palm up.

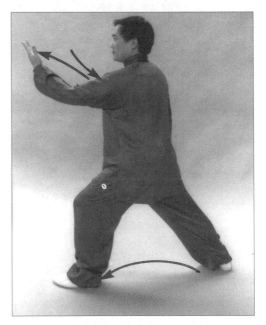

Step forward with your left foot, touching down with your heel first. Begin turning your body to your left while pulling your right hand down and extending your left hand forward.

Posture 22: High Pat on Horse (Gao Tan Ma)

Movements

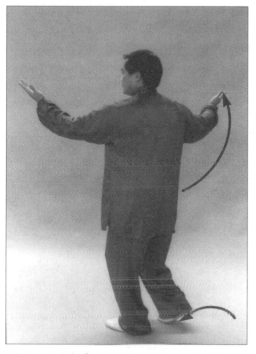

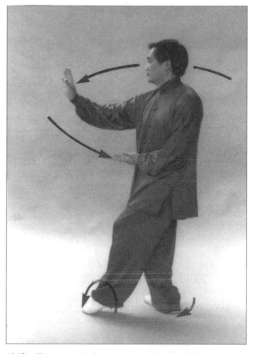

Bring your right foot a half step forward while extending your right palm back, palm up.

Shift all your weight to your right leg, lift your left foot slightly, and touch down on the ball of your left foot. At the same time, bend your right elbow and extend your right palm forward while pulling your left palm back next to your waist.

Posture 23: Right Heel Kick (You Deng Jiao)

Movements

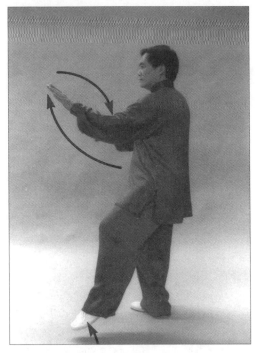

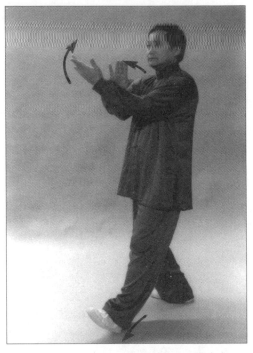

Lift up your left foot while you circle your left palm up and lower your right palm next to your left elbow. Both palms face down.

Step to your upper left corner with your left foot. At the same time, bring your left arm in slightly, rotating your left palm until it faces you, while extending your right palm over your left wrist. (Step southwest.)

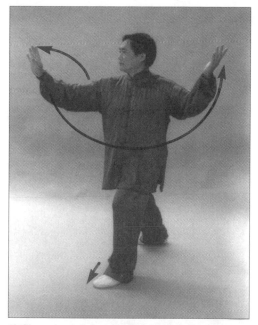

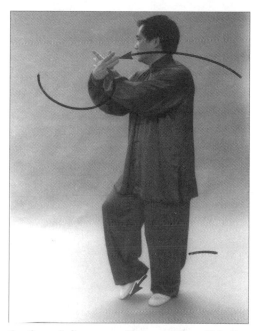

Shift your weight to your left leg into bow stance. At the same time, circle your right palm up and to your right, and circle your left palm down and to your left.

Continue circling your palms up and in until both palms are crossed in front of you, right palm touching the outside of your left wrist.

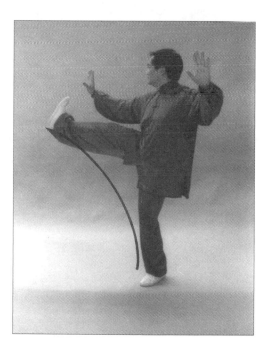

Extend both palms to your sides while kicking to your right with the heel of your right foot. (Kick northwest.)

Posture 24: Strike to Ears with Both Fists (Shuang Feng Guan Er)

Movements

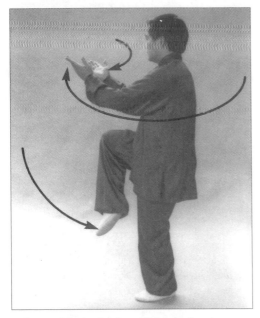

Pull your right leg back and bring both palms together until your palms are facing you.

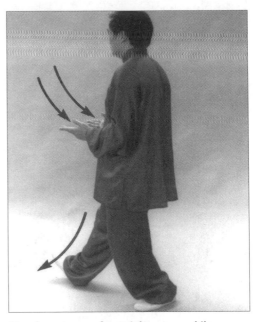

Step down to your front right corner while lowering your palms next to your abdomen.

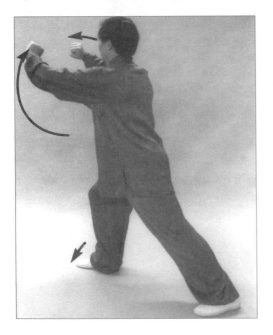

Change your palms to fists and circle both fists to your sides and then up. Palms of your fists face forward. Shift your weight forward to your right foot and bring your fists closer together.

Posture 25: Left Heel Kick (Zuo Deng Jiao)

Movements

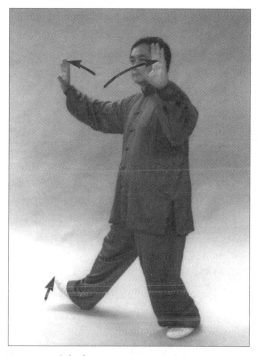 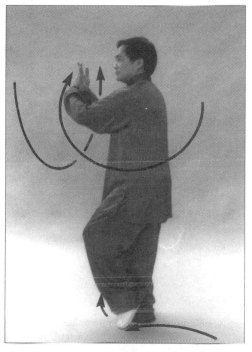

Turn your right foot out to your right. Open your fists and separate your palms to your sides.

Shift all your weight on your right foot and bring your left foot next to your right one while circling both palms down until they cross and the palms face you, left palm on the outside. As you lift up your left foot, rotate both palms until they face forward. Then begin to separate your palms to the sides.

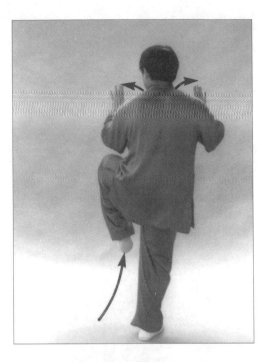

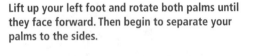

Lift up your left foot and rotate both palms until they face forward. Then begin to separate your palms to the sides.

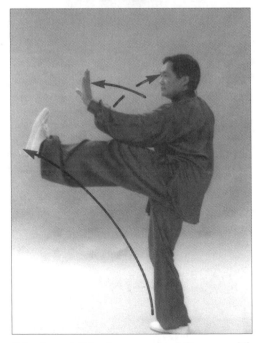

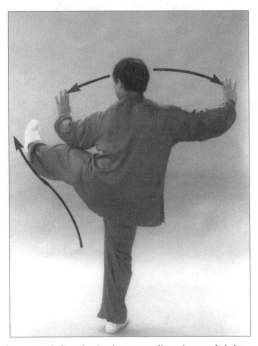

Extend your left leg to your upper left corner while extending your left palm in the same direction and right palm to your right. (See rear view. Kick northwest.)

Posture 26: Cover Hand and Strike with Fist (Yan Shou Liao Quan)

Movements

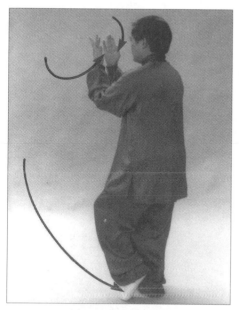

Lower your left foot and touch the ball of the left foot next to your right foot while you bring both forearms next to each other, palms facing you.

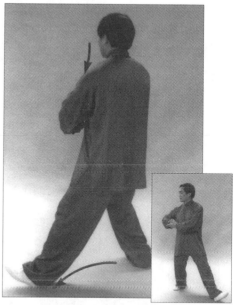

Step to your upper left corner with your left foot while lowering both arms. Right hand is held in a fist and placed on top of your left palm. (See front view. Step southwest.)

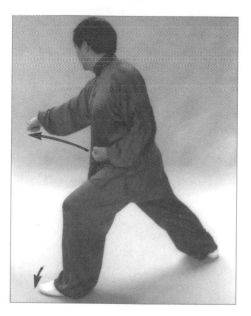

Shift your weight to your left leg into bow stance. At the same time, *pull your left hand back to your waist in a fist and whip your right fist out in front of you.* (*Quick Tempo*) (Face northwest.)

Posture 27: Needle at Sea Bottom (Haidi Zhen)

Movements

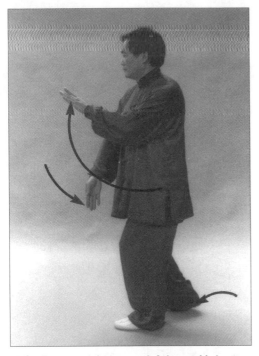 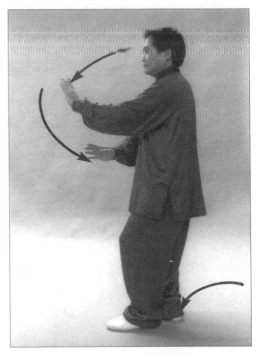

Shift all your weight to your left leg and bring your right foot a half step up behind your left foot. At the same time, open both fists, lower your right palm, and circle your left palm up.

Shift your weight to your right foot. At the same time, bring your left palm forward and down. The right palm begins to circle backward.

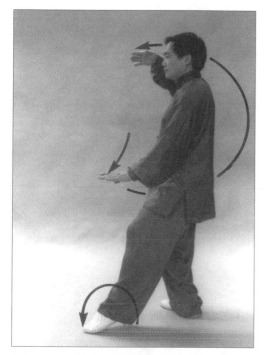

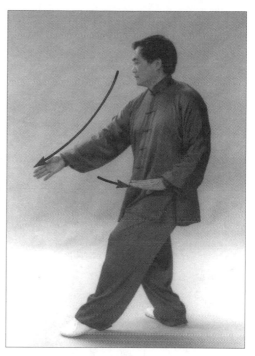

Lift up your left foot slightly off the floor and circle your right hand back and up until it is next to your ear. Palm is facing inward.

Pull your left palm toward your waist, touch down on your left foot, and spear down with your right palm. (Face west.)

Posture 28: Fan Through Back (Shan Tong Bei)

Movements

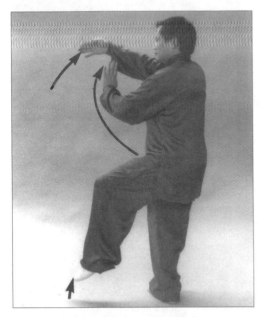

Lift up both palms, left fingers just below your right wrist, while lifting up your left foot slightly.

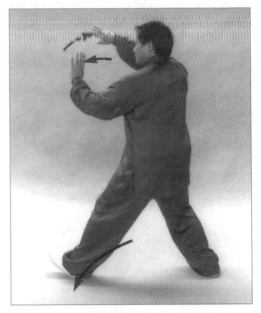

Step forward with your left foot, and begin pulling your right palm back and extending your left palm forward.

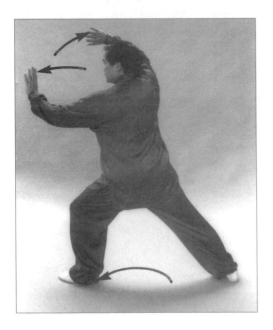

Shift your weight forward into left bow stance, pull your right palm over your head, and extend your left palm in front of you.

SECTION V

Posture 29: Right and Left Toe Kick (Zuo You Fen Jiao)

Movements

Toe Kick, right side

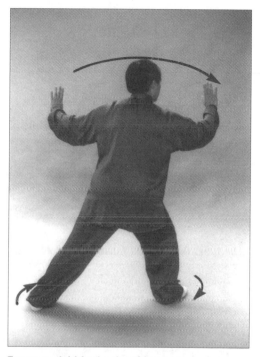 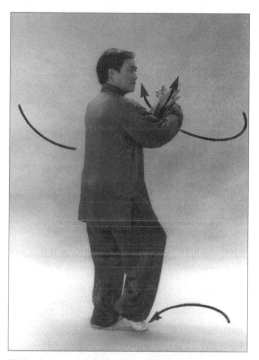

Turn your right foot out and turn your body around, 180 degrees. At the same time, lower your right palm to your right.

Shift all your weight back to your left leg and touch the ball of your right foot next to your left foot. At the same time, circle both palms down and up until they are crossed in front of your body. Both palms face you with the inside of your right wrist touching the outside of your left wrist. (Face east.)

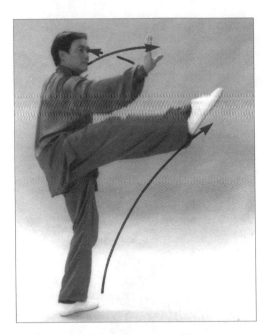

Lift your right knee and kick up with your right foot toward your upper right corner. At the same time, extend your right arm in the direction of your kick and extend your left arm to your left. (Kick southeast.)

Toe Kick, left side

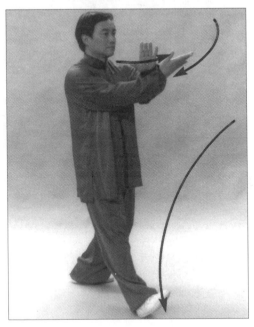

Bring your foot down in the direction of your kick. At the same time, lower your right forearm and bring your left palm across your right arm. (Step southeast.)

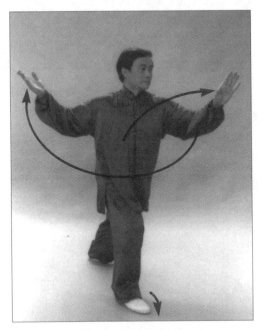

Shift your weight to your right leg into bow stance while circling and extending your left palm to your left and circling your right palm down and up to your right.

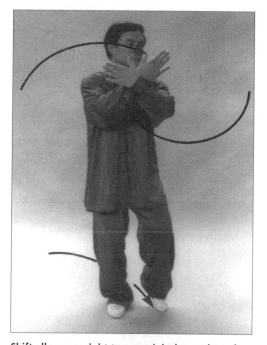

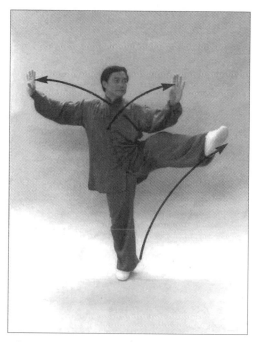

Shift all your weight to your right leg and touch the ball of your left foot next to your right foot. At the same time, continue the circular movements of your palms until they are crossed next to your body. The inside of your left wrist touches the outside of your right wrist.

Lift your left knee and kick up with your left foot toward your upper left corner. At the same time, extend your left arm in the direction of your kick and extend your right arm to your right. (Kick northeast.)

Posture 30: Brush Knee and Step Forward (Lou Xi Ao Bu)

Movements

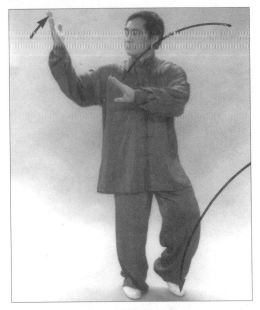

Lower your left foot next to your right foot. At the same time, bend your right elbow and bring your left palm in front of your right armpit.

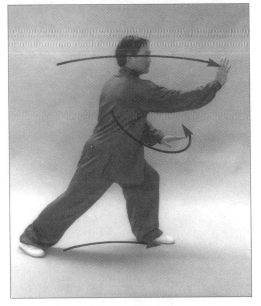

Step forward with your left foot and shift your weight onto it into the bow stance. Extend your right palm forward.

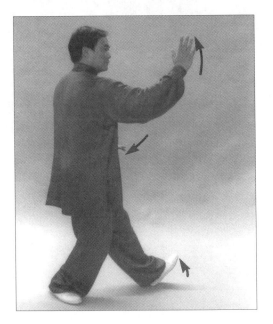

Shift your weight back to your right foot. Turn your left foot outward and begin turning your body to your left while rotating your right palm inward and pulling your left palm next to your abdomen.

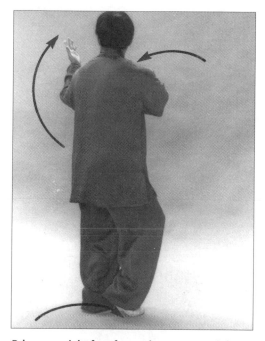

Bring your right foot forward next to your left one while circling your left arm up to head level, and begin lowering your right palm, face down.

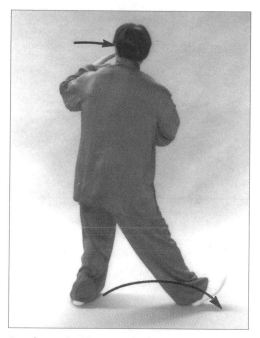

Step forward with your right foot while beginning to brush your right palm across your right knee, and extend your left palm forward.

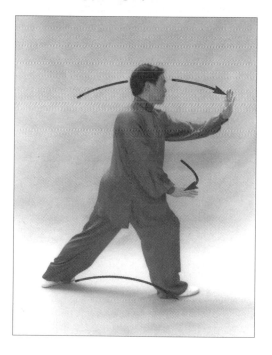

Shift your weight to your right foot into bow stance and extend your left palm forward.

Posture 31: Step Forward, Grab, and Punch (Shang Bu Qin Da)

Movements

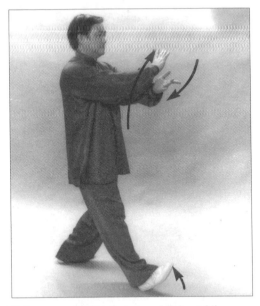

Shift your weight back to your left leg while extending your right forearm over your left forearm.

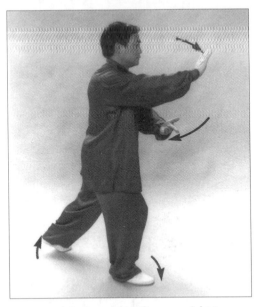

Turn your right foot out, shift your weight to your right leg, and begin to step forward with your left foot. At the same time, circle your right palm forward and lower your left palm.

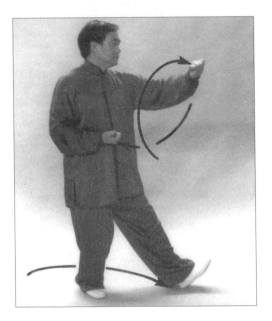

Step forward with your left leg while pulling your right hand back to your waist in a fist and circling your left hand forward in a fist.

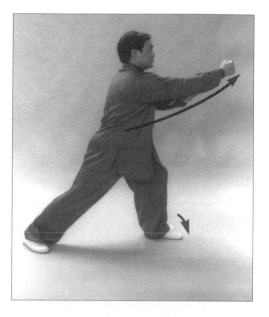

Shift your weight forward into bow stance while punching forward with your right fist.

Posture 32: Appears Closed (Ru Feng Si Bi)

Movements

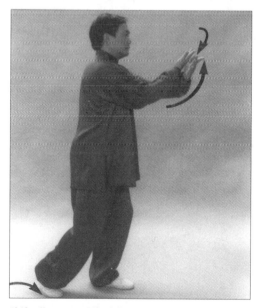

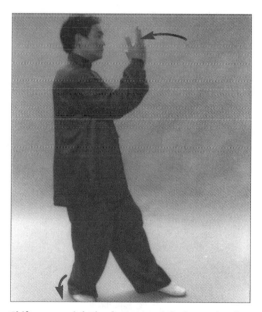

Shift all your weight forward to your left leg and bring your right foot half a step forward behind your left foot. At the same time, open your fists and extend your right palm over your left forearm. Both palms rotate in.

Shift your weight back to your right leg and pull your palms in closer to your face.

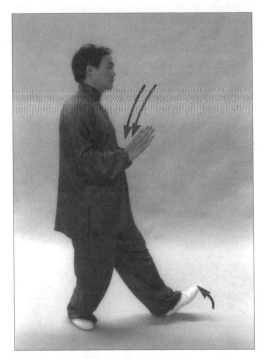

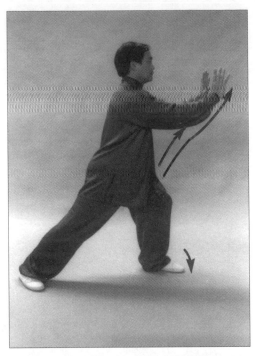

Rotate, separate, and lower your palms until your palms are facing down and next to your abdomen.

Push forward with both palms while shifting your weight to your left foot into bow stance.

Posture 33: Left Wave Hands Like Clouds (Zuo Yun Shou)

Movements

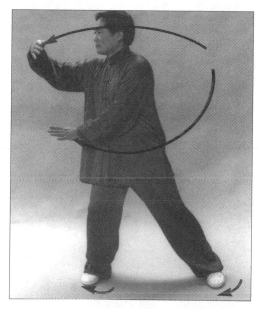

Turn your right foot out and turn your body to your right while pulling your right palm across your face and lowering your left palm to your right.

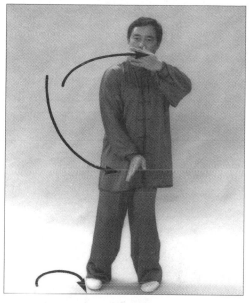

Circle your left palm up while lowering your right hand and moving your right foot closer to your left foot.

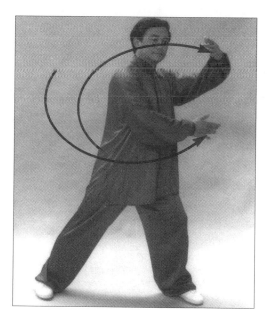

Step toward your left with your left foot. Circle your left palm across your face while lowering your left palm and circling it to your left.

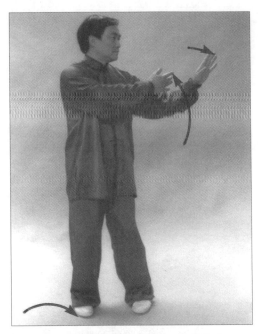

Move your right foot closer to your left foot. Continue with the previous palm movements, lowering your left palm and lifting your right palm.

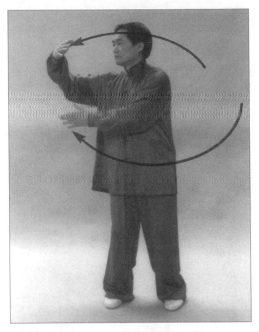

Turn your waist to your right while circling your right palm up and across your face and lowering your left palm.

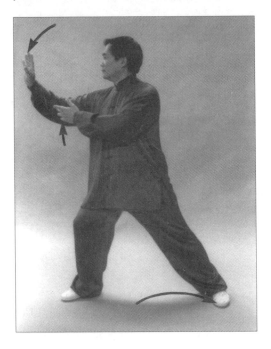

Step to your left with your left foot while extending your right palm to the side, palm down, and begin lifting up your left palm.

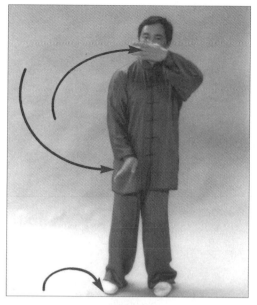

Continue circling your left palm up while lowering your right hand and moving your right foot closer to your left foot.

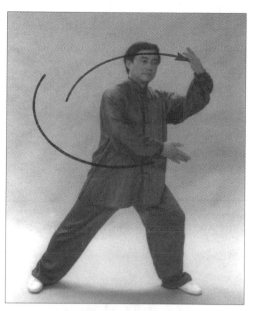

Step toward your left with your left foot. Continue circling your left palm across your face while lowering your right hand.

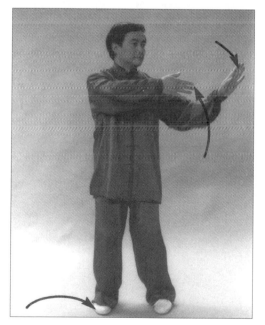

Move your right foot closer to your left foot. Continue with the previous palm movements, lowering your left palm and lifting your right palm.

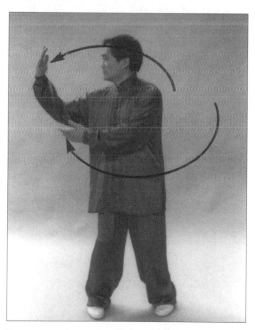

Turn your waist to your right while circling your right palm up and across your face and lowering your left palm.

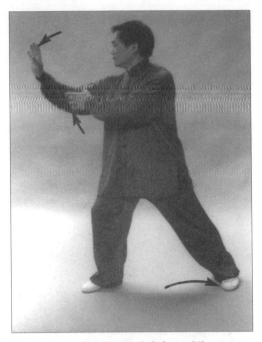

Step to your left with your left foot while extending your right palm to the side, palm down, and begin lifting up your left palm.

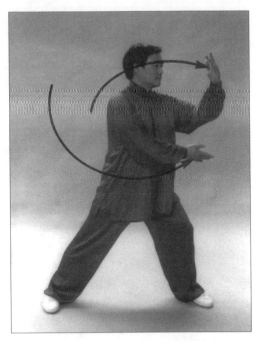

Continue circling your left palm up and across your face while lowering your right hand.

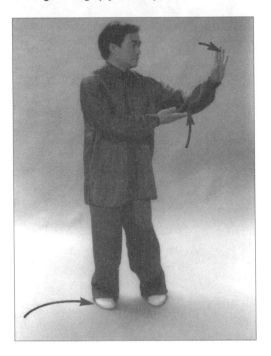

Move your right foot closer to your left foot. Continue with the previous palm movements, lowering your left palm and lifting your right palm.

Posture 34: Right Diagonal Back Fist (You Pie Shen Chui)

Movements

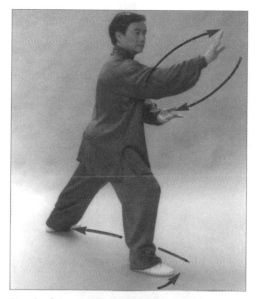

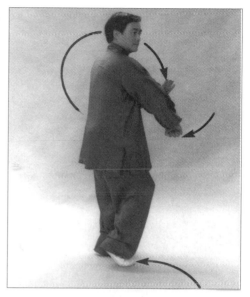

Step back to your back left corner with your left foot into bow stance. At the same time, extend your right palm over your left palm while pulling your left palm next to your body. Right palm faces forward and left palm faces up. (Step northwest.)

Shift your weight to your left leg and touch the ball of your right foot next to your left foot. At the same time, lower both arms and bring your left palm on top of your right forearm with right hand held in a fist.

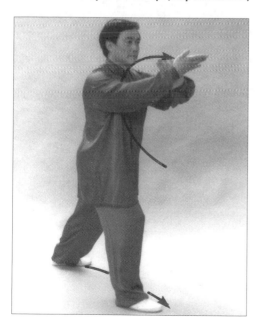

Step forward to your upper right corner into bow stance and circle your right fist up and forward. Left hand maintains contact with your right forearm. (Step southeast.)

Posture 35: Left and Right Shuttle Back and Forth (Zuo You Chuan Suo)

Movements

Shuttle Back and Forth, left side

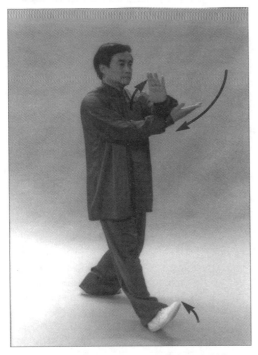

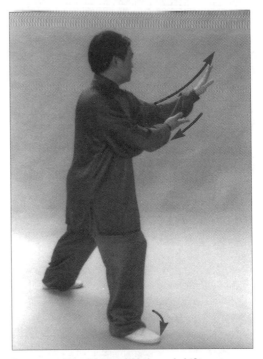

Shift your weight back to your left leg and lift up the ball of your right foot. At the same time, open your right hand and extend your left palm over your right forearm.

Turn your right foot in slightly and shift your weight forward into bow stance. At the same time, pull your right palm in closer to your body and circle your left palm forward.

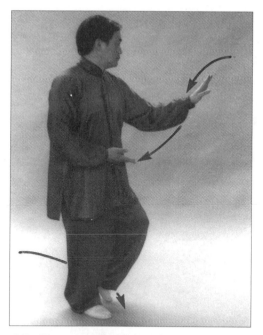

Shift all your weight to your right leg and touch the ball of your left foot next to your right one. At the same time, begin lowering both palms.

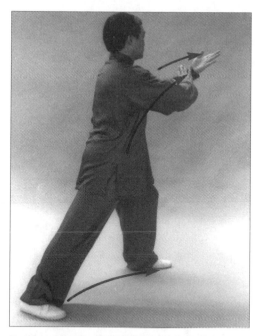

Continue lowering both palms down, and then up to chest level. Touch your right palm on your left wrist. Then step to your upper left corner with your left foot into bow stance while you extend both palms forward. (Step northeast.)

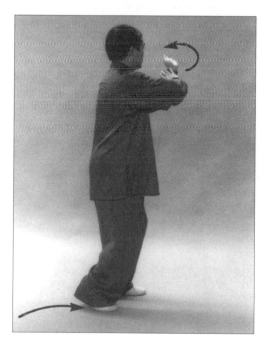

Shift all your weight forward and touch the ball of your right foot next to your left foot. At the same time, begin making a horizontal circle to your left with your left palm.

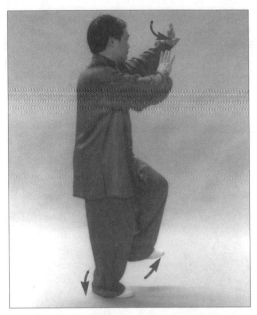

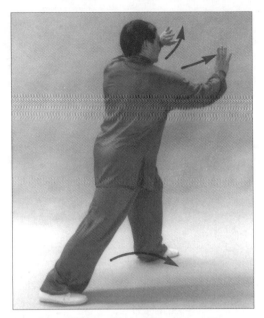

Shift all your weight to your right leg and lift your left foot off the floor while completing the horizontal circle with your left palm.

Step forward to your upper left corner with your left foot into bow stance. At the same time, raise your left forearm and extend your right palm forward. (Step northeast.)

Shuttle Back and Forth, right side

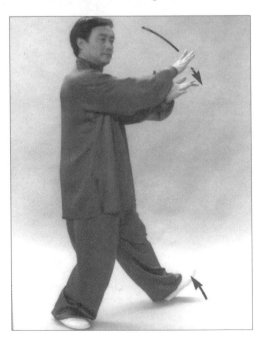

Shift your weight back to your right leg and lower your left arm. At the same time, extend your right palm over your left forearm.

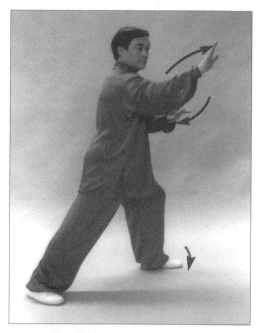

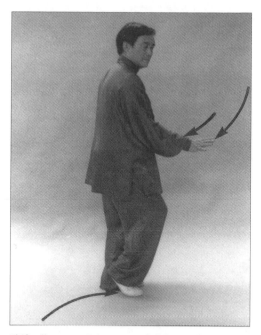

Turn your left foot in slightly and shift your weight forward into bow stance. At the same time, pull your left palm in closer to your body and circle your right palm forward.

Shift all your weight to your left leg and touch the ball of your right foot next to your left foot. At the same time, lower both palms to waist level.

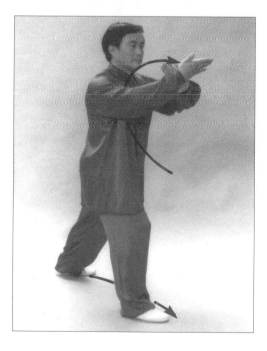

Continue lowering both palms down, and then up to chest level. Touch your left palm on your right wrist. Then step to your upper right corner with your right foot into bow stance while you extend both palms forward. (Step southeast.)

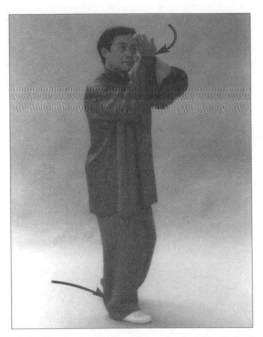

Shift all your weight forward and touch the ball of your left foot next to your right foot. At the same time, begin making a horizontal circle to your right with your right palm.

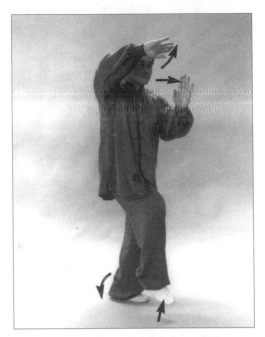

Shift all your weight to your left leg and lift your right foot off the floor while completing the horizontal circle with your right palm.

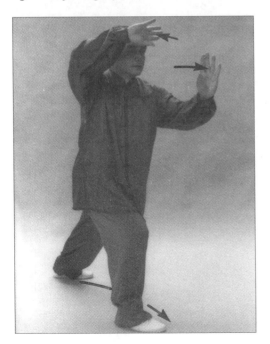

Step forward to your upper right corner with your right foot into bow stance. At the same time, raise your right forearm and extend your left palm forward. (Step southeast.)

Posture 36: Step Back and Spear Palm (Tui Bu Chuan Zhang)

Movements

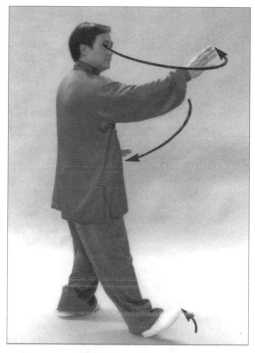

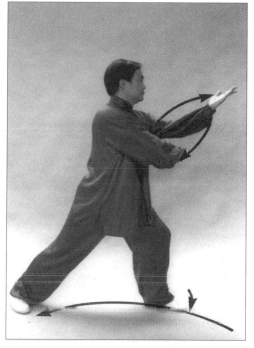

Shift your weight back to your left leg while lowering your right palm to chest level and lowering your left palm next to your waist.

Step back with your right foot behind you into bow stance. At the same time, pull your right palm closer to your body while spearing your left palm over your right forearm. Rotate your left palm up as you spear forward. (Step west. Face east.)

SECTION VI

Posture 37: Insubstantial Stance and Press Palm Down (Xu Bu Ya Zhang)

Movements

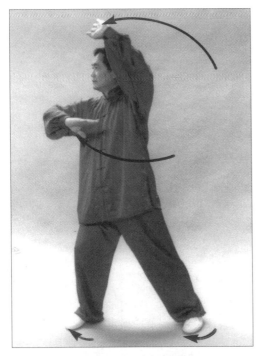

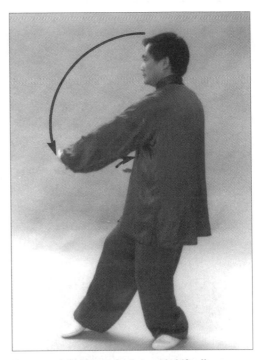

Turn your right foot out and left foot in as you turn your body 180 degrees to your back. At the same time, raise your left forearm over your head.

Turn your left foot in farther and shift all your weight on it. At the same time, pull your right palm down next to your waist and press your left palm down. (Face west.)

Posture 38: Stand on One Leg and Lift Palm (Du Li Tuo Zhang)

Movements

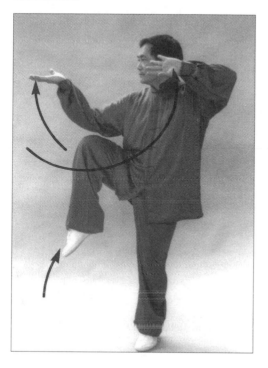

Lift your right knee and straighten your left leg. At the same time, pull your left palm up to ear level and lift your right palm up in front of you at shoulder level.

Posture 39: Lean in Horse Stance (Ma Bu Kao)

Movements

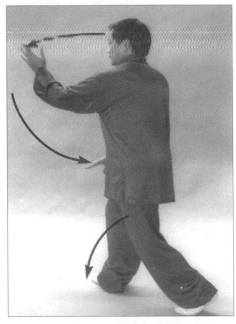

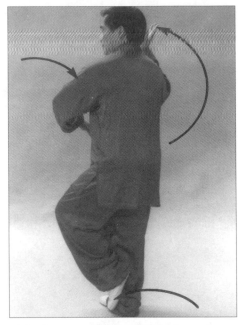

Step down in front of you with your right foot turned out, and shift all your weight on it. At the same time, extend your left palm forward and pull your right palm down next to your waist.

Shift all your weight to your right leg and touch the ball of your left foot next to your right. At the same time, circle your right palm back and up to ear level, palm facing forward, and lower your left palm next to your body, palm facing down.

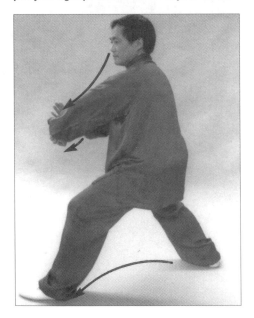

Step to your upper left corner with your left foot. At the same time, place your right hand on top of your left wrist with your left hand held in a fist. *Then press your left forearm and right palm down at an angle together.* (*Quick Tempo*) (Step southwest.)

Posture 40: Turn Body and Large Rollback (Zhuan Shen Da Lu)

Movements

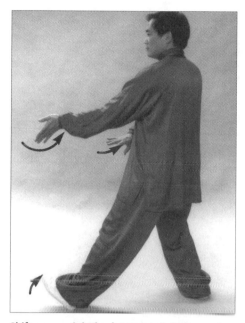

Shift your weight back to your right leg and separate your arms. Right palm faces down and left palm faces up at an angle.

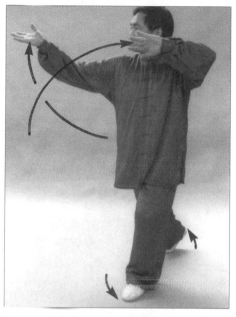

Turn your left foot out and shift your weight on it. At the same time, pull your left palm up to ear level and lift up your right palm in front of you at shoulder level.

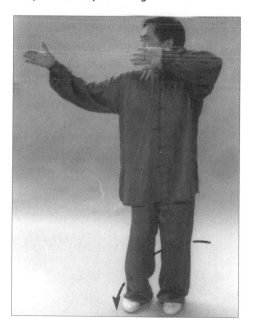

*Bring your right foot next to your left foot and stand up.

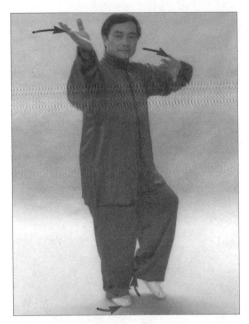

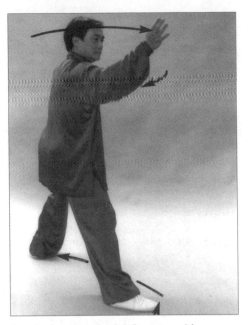

Turn your right foot in and shift all your weight to your right leg while lifting up your left heel. At the same time, begin pulling your palms down to your left.* (* *Quick Tempo*)

Step back to your back left corner with your left foot and continue to lower your palms. Both palms face to your left. (Step northwest.)

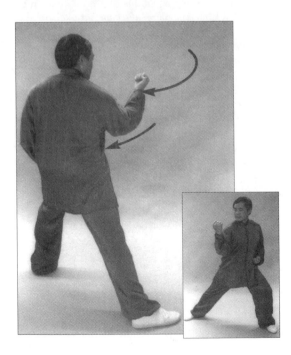

Bring your left hand next to your waist, with that hand held in a fist. At the same time, lower your right arm in front of your body with that hand held in a fist. (See front view. Face northeast.)

Posture 41: Scoop Palm and Lower Body (Liao Zhang Xia Shi)

Movements

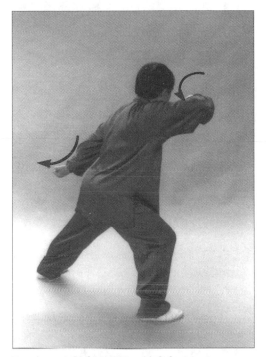 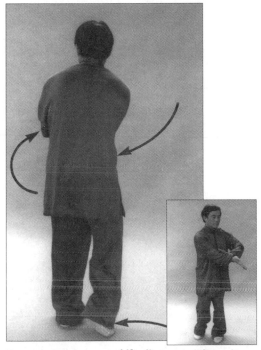

Turn your right foot out and left foot in as you shift your weight forward to your right leg into bow stance. At the same time, extend your right elbow to your right and coil your left fist down to your left. The right fist is next to your head, facing down; the left fist is facing up.

Turn your left foot out, shift all your weight on it, and touch the ball of your right foot next to your left foot. At the same time, open both fists, circle your left palm clockwise up, and scoop your right palm down and forward. The left palm is on top of your right forearm. (See front view. Face northwest.)

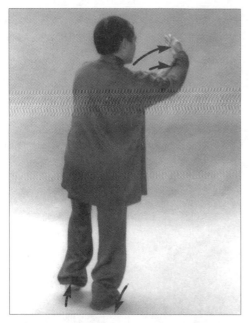

Shift all your weight to your right leg and lift up your left heel. Lift up both palms to your right with your left palm maintaining contact with your right forearm.

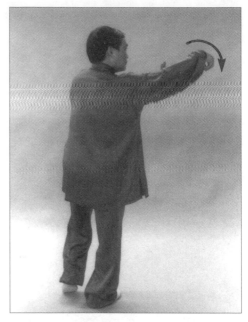

Extend your right arm to your right and hook your hand down.

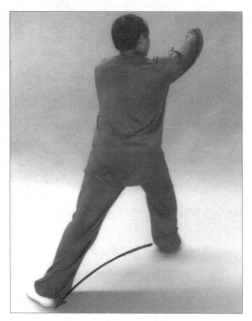

Step to your back left corner with your left foot. (Step southwest.)

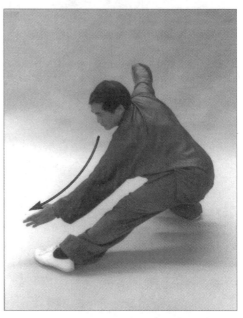

Lower your body and extend your left palm along the inside of your left leg until it is next to your left foot.

Posture 42: Step Forward and Cross Punch (Shang Bu Shi Zi Quan)

Movements

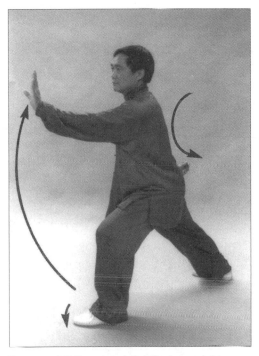

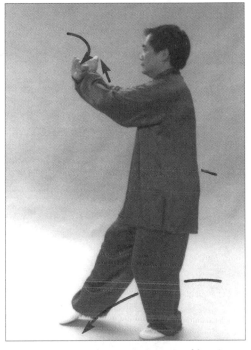

Turn your left foot out and shift your weight forward. At the same time, lift up your left palm, lower your right arm, and turn your right hand up in a hook.

Step forward with your right foot, touching down on the ball of your right foot. At the same time, hold both hands in fists, bring your left arm in closer to your body, and extend your right fist forward until it is next to your left fist. The right fist faces forward and the left fist faces in. (Face west.)

Posture 43: Stand on One Leg and Ride the Tiger (Du Li Kua Hu)

Movements

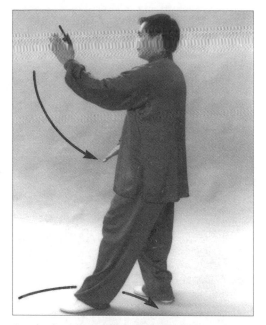

Step back with your right foot and shift your weight on it. At the same time, open both palms and lower your right palm next to your waist.

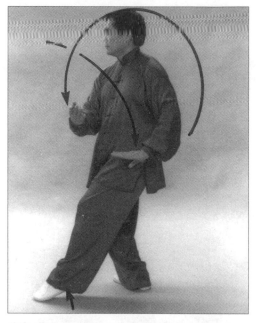

Shift all your weight to your right leg and begin lifting up your left foot. At the same time, pull your left palm down next to your waist, circle your right palm back and up, and then down in front of your body.

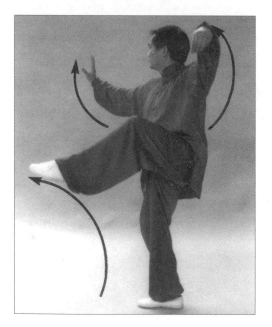

Lift up your left foot in front of you. At the same time, lift up your right palm in front of you, extending your left arm up and to your left, as you change the palm into a hook.

Posture 44: Turn Body and Sweep Lotus (Zhuan Shen Bai Lian)

Movements

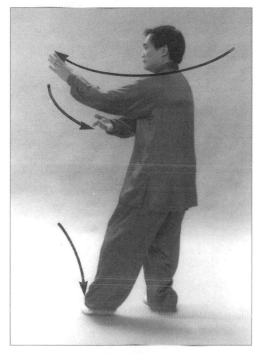

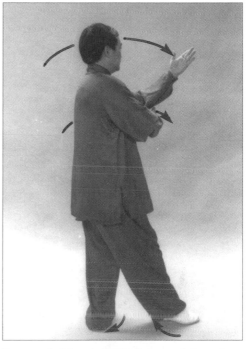

Lower your left foot in front of you. At the same time, open your left palm, swing it around until it is in front of you, and lower your right palm until it is under your left elbow.

Turn your left foot in, shift all your weight on it, and turn your right foot out. At the same time, turn your body to your right. Left palm rotates in with your body until it faces up at an angle.

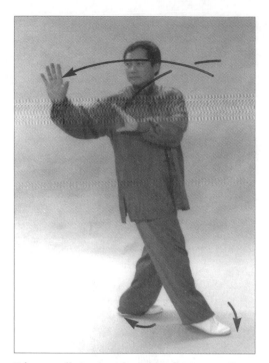

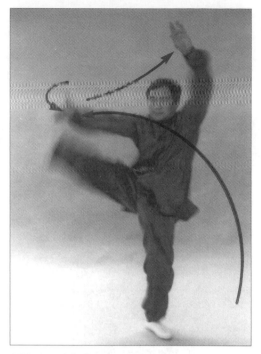

Take a small step to your right and turn your foot out while extending both palms to your right.

Lift your right leg up and sweep it across your face while slapping both palms across your right foot and pulling your hands to your left. (*Quick Tempo*) (Face south. Kick from east to west.)

Posture 45: Pull the Bow and Shoot the Tiger (Wan Gong She Hu)

Movements

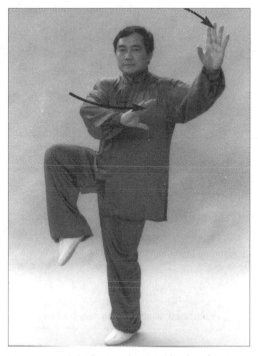

Lower your right foot and extend both palms to your left.

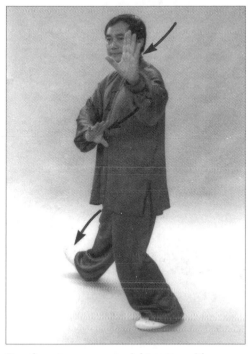

Step down to your upper right corner with your right foot and begin to lower both palms. (Step northwest.)

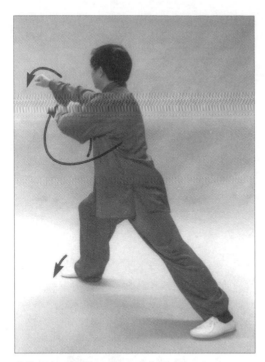

Shift your weight to your right leg into bow stance while continuing to lower your palms down and then up to your right. Left arm is bent, with both hands held in fists.

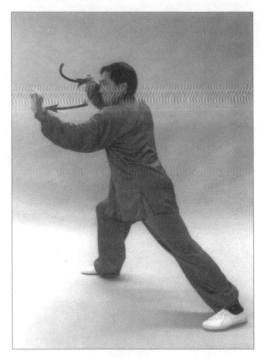

Turn your head to your left while extending your left fist to your left and lifting your right forearm to forehead level. Left fist faces up. (Face southwest.)

Posture 46: Right Deflect, Parry, and Punch (You Ban Lan Chui)

Movements

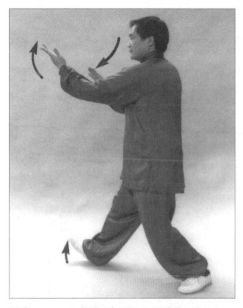

Shift your weight back to your left leg. At the same time, open both fists, rotate your left palm up, and extend your right palm next to your left forearm. Right palm faces down.

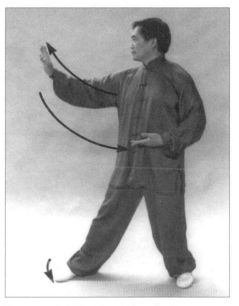

Turn your right foot in while extending your right palm forward and pulling your left palm next to your waist.

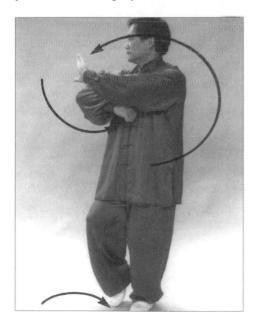

Shift all your weight to your left leg and touch the ball of your right foot next to your left foot. At the same time, hold your right hand into a fist and lower your right forearm next to your chest and circle your left palm in.

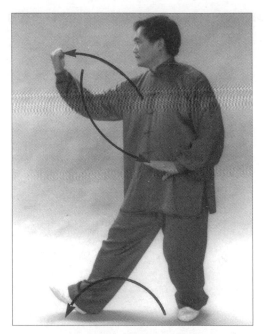

Step forward with your right foot while circling your right fist forward and pulling your left palm down next to your waist. (Step west.)

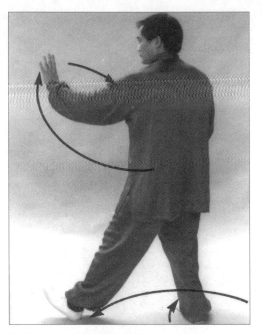

Shift your weight forward to your right leg, turn your foot out, and step forward with your left foot. At the same time, extend your left palm forward and pull your right fist back to your waist, facing up.

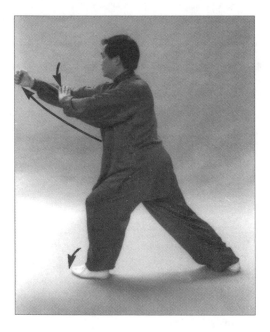

Shift your weight forward into bow stance while punching forward with your right fist.

Posture 47: Right Wardoff, Rollback, Press, and Push (You Peng Lu Ji An)

Movements

Wardoff, right side

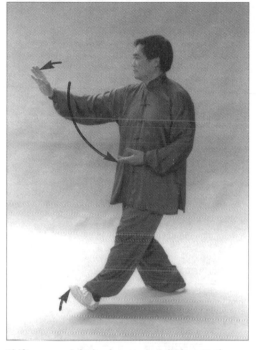

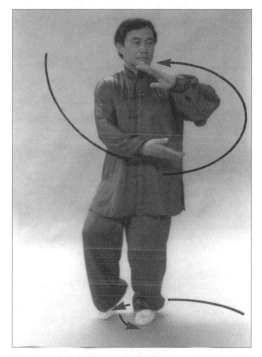

Shift your weight back to your right leg. At the same time, open your right fist and pull your left hand back to your waist with palm facing up.

Turn your left foot out, shift all your weight on it, and touch the ball of your right foot next to your left foot.

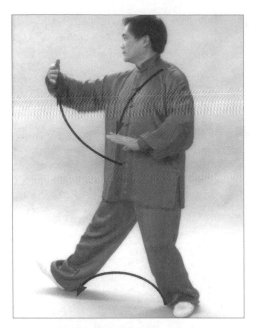

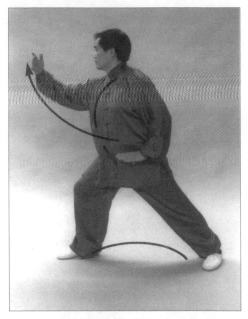

Step forward with your right foot and touch down with your heel first while beginning to extend your right forearm forward and pulling your left palm down.

Shift your weight forward into a right bow stance and complete the previous arm movements. This is the completion of the right wardoff posture.

Rollback, right side

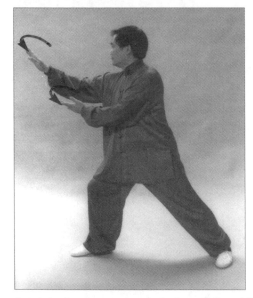

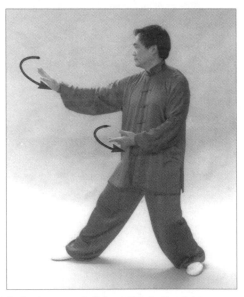

Rotate both palms counterclockwise and then shift your weight back to your left foot. This is the right rollback posture.

Press, right side

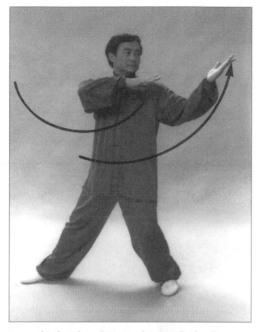

Lower both palms down and up to the back.

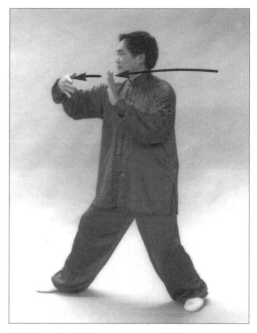

Continue the circular movements of your arms and begin extending them forward.

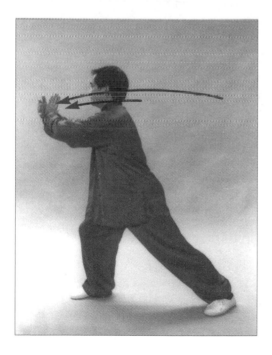

Touch your left palm to your right wrist and extend both palms forward while shifting your weight to your right foot. This is the completion of the right press posture.

Push, right side

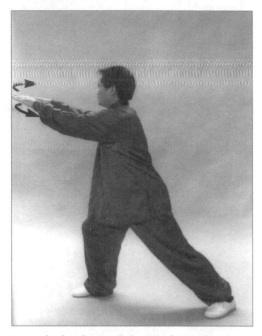

Rotate both palms until they are facing down.

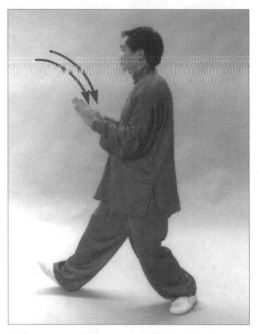

Shift your weight to your left foot. Pull both palms in and down to your abdomen.

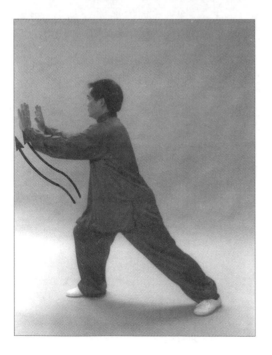

Push forward with both palms while shifting your weight to your right foot. This is the completion of the right push posture.

Posture 48: Cross Hands (Shi Zi Shou)

Movements

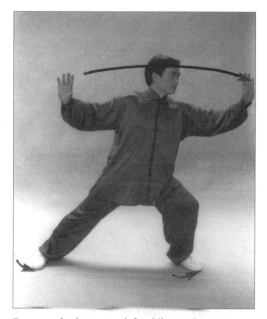

Turn your body to your left while turning your left foot out and right foot in. At the same time, extend your left arm to your left.

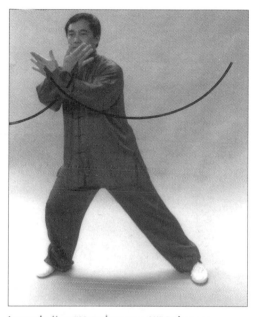

Lower both arms and scoop your palms up, crossing them in front of your chest.

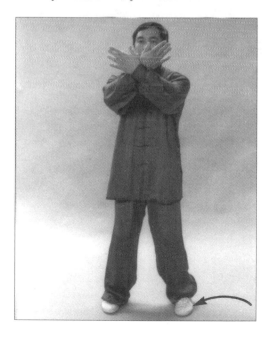

Shift your weight to your right leg and bring your left foot closer in until both feet are shoulder width apart. (Face south.)

Closing (Shou Shi)

Movements

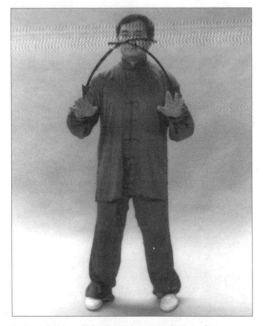

Rotate both palms until they are facing down.

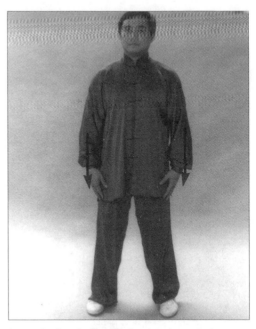

Lower both palms to hip level and stand up completely.

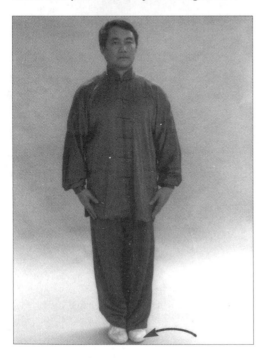

Bring your left foot next to your right and relax, hands down to your sides.

Acknowledgements

Special Thanks (in alphabetical order):

Carol Shearer-Best, for her valuable suggestions and proofreading
Joseph Best, Jr., for his valuable suggestions and proofreading
Deborah Clark, for her cover design for the 1995 edition
Reza Farman-Farmaian, for his photography
Jerry Leake, for graphic design and typesetting of the 1995 edition
James O'Leary, for his valuable suggestions and proofreading
Jeff Pratt, for his valuable suggestions and proofreading
David Ripianzi, for his suggestions with publication
Ramel Rones, for his valuable comments
William Walker, his valuable ideas and the use of his reference books
Roger Whidden, for his valuable suggestions and proofreading
Dr. Yang, Jwing-Ming, for his technical advice

Movement Names for the 24 and 48 Postures

24 Posture Taijiquan (Ershisi Shi Taijiquan)

Simplified Taijiquan (Jianhua Taijiquan)

1. Commencing (Qi Shi)
2. The Wild Horse Parts Its Mane (Ye Ma Fen Zong)
3. White Crane Spreads Its Wings (Bai He Liang Chi)
4. Brush Knee and Step Forward (Lou Xi Ao Bu)
5. Playing the Lute (Shou Hui Pipa)
6. Reverse Reeling Forearm (Dao Juan Gong)
7. Left Grasp Sparrow's Tail (Zuo Lan Que Wei)
8. Right Grasp Sparrow's Tail (You Lan Que Wei)
9. Single Whip (Dan Bian)
10. Wave Hands Like Clouds (Yun Shou)
11. Single Whip (Dan Bian)
12. High Pat on Horse (Gao Tan Ma)
13. Right Heel Kick (You Deng Jiao)
14. Strike to Ears with Both Fists (Shuang Feng Guan Er)
15. Turn Body and Left Heel Kick (Zhuan Shen Zuo Deng Jiao)
16. Left Lower Body and Stand on One Leg (Zuo Xia Shi Du Li)
17. Right Lower Body and Stand on One Leg (You Xia Shi Du Li)
18. Shuttle Back and Forth (Chuan Suo)
19. Needle at Sea Bottom (Haidi Zhen)
20. Fan through Back (Shan Tong Bei)
21. Turn Body, Deflect, Parry, and Punch (Zhuan Shen Ban Lan Chui)

22. Appears Closed (Ru Feng Si Bi)

23. Cross Hands (Shi Zi Shou)

24. Closing (Shou Shi)

48 Posture Taijiquan (Sishiba Shi Taijiquan)

Commencing (Qi Shi)

1. White Crane Spreads Its Wings (Bai He Liang Chi)

2. Left Brush Knee and Step Forward (Zuo Lou Xi Ao Bu)

3. Left Single Whip (Zuo Dan Bian)

4. Left Lute Posture (Zuo Pipa Shi)

5. Rollback and Press Posture (Lu Ji Shi)

6. Left Deflect, Parry, and Punch (Zuo Ban Lan Chui)

7. Left Wardoff, Rollback, Press, and Push (Zuo Peng Lu Ji An)

8. Lean on a Diagonal (Xie Shen Kao)

9. Fist under Elbow (Zhou Di Chui)

10. Reverse Reeling Forearm (Dao Juan Gong)

11. Turn Body and Thrust Palm (Zhuan Shen Tui Zhang)

12. Right Lute Posture (You Pipa Shi)

13. Brush Knee and Punch Down (Lou Xi Cai Chui)

14. White Snake Spits Poison (Bai She Tu Xin)

15. Slap Foot and Tame the Tiger (Pai Jiao Fu Hu)

16. Left Diagonal Backfist (Zuo Pie Shen Chui)

17. Piercing Fist and Lower Body (Chuanquan Xia Shi)

18. Stand on One Leg and Prop Up Palm (Du Li Cheng Zhang)

19. Right Single Whip (You Dan Bian)

20. Right Wave Hands Like Clouds (You Yun Shou)

21. Left and Right The Wild Horse Parts Its Mane (Zuo You Fen Zong)

22. High Pat on Horse (Gao Tan Ma)

23. Right Heel Kick (You Deng Jiao)

24. Strike to Ears with Both Fists (Shuang Feng Guan Er)

25. Left Heel Kick (Zuo Deng Jiao)
26. Cover Hand and Strike with Fist (Yan Shou Liao Quan)
27. Needle at Sea Bottom (Haidi Zhen)
28. Fan through Back (Shan Tong Bei)
29. Right and Left Toe Kick (Zuo You Fen Jiao)
30. Brush Knee and Step Forward (Lou Xi Ao Bu)
31. Step Forward, Grab, and Punch (Shang Bu Qin Da)
32. Appears Closed (Ru Feng Si Bi)
33. Left Wave Hands Like Clouds (Zuo Yun Shou)
34. Right Diagonal Backfist (You Pie Shen Chui)
35. Left and Right Shuttle Back and Forth (Zuo You Chuan Suo)
36. Step Back and Spear Palm (Tui Bu Chuan Zhang)
37. Insubstantial Stance and Press Palm Down (Xu Bu Ya Zhang)
38. Stand on One Leg and Lift Palm (Du Li Tuo Zhang)
39. Lean in Horse Stance (Ma Bu Kao)
40. Turn Body and Large Rollback (Zhuan Shen Da Lu)
41. Scoop Palm and Lower Body (Liao Zhang Xia Shi)
42. Step Forward and Cross Punch (Shang Bu Shi Zi Quan)
43. Stand on One Leg and Ride the Tiger (Du Li Kua Hu)
44. Turn Body and Sweep Lotus (Zhuan Shen Bai Lian)
45. Pull the Bow and Shoot the Tiger (Wan Gong She Hu)
46. Right Deflect, Parry, and Punch (You Ban Lan Chui)
47. Right Wardoff, Rollback, Press, and Push (You Peng Lu Ji An)
48. Cross Hands (Shi Zi Shou)

Closing (Shou Shi)

GLOSSARY

Baguazhang. An internal Chinese martial arts style.

baihui. An acupuncture cavity on top of the head.

Beijing (Peking). Capital city of the People's Republic of China.

bianshi. Stone probe used for acupuncture in ancient China.

Chen Style. One of the five major taijiquan styles.

Chen, Chang-xing. Fourteenth-generation Chen descendant who taught Yang, Lu-chan taijiquan (AD 1771–1853).

chen jian chuiz hou. Sink the shoulders and drop the elbows.

Chen, Qing-ping. A student of Chen, You-ben; creator of a variation of Chen Style Taijiquan called Zhaobao Style (AD 1795–1868).

Chen, Wang-ting. One of the legendary founders of taijiquan.

Chen, Yan-lin. Author of *Taijiquan, Saber, Sword, Staff, and Sparring*.

Chen, You-ben. Fourteenth-generation Chen descendant, created a variation of the Chen Style Taijiquan called New Frame Style.

Chen, Yu-ting. Another name for Chen, Wang-ting.

Chenjiagou. Chen Family Village.

dan tian (dan dien). An acupuncture cavity below the navel.

Dao qi ling he. Guiding the qi to achieve harmony.

Dao yin. Guiding and stretching.

Daoist (Taoist). A person who follows the philosophy of Daoism.

Dapeng Qigong. A style of qigong.

dian qi. Electric energy.

Emei Mountain. A mountain in China.

fen qing xu shi. Distinguish substantial and insubstantial.

Feng, Yi-yuan. Legendary teacher of Zhang, San-feng.

gong bu. Bow stance.

gou. Hand hook.

guan qi fa. Qi permeating technique.

ha. Sound emitted during practice.

han xiong ba bei. Arc your chest and round your back.

He, Wei-zhen. Student of Li, Yi-yu; teacher of Sun, Lu-tang (AD 1849–1920).

Hebei. A province in southern China.

Henan. A province in China.

heng. Sound emitted during practice.

Hua Tuo. Creator and author of *Five Animal Play*.

hou tian fa. Post-heaven techniques.

Hua Mountain. A mountain in Shaanxi Province, China.

Huang, Li-zhou. Author of *Wangzhongnan Muzhiming*.

Huangdi Neijing. *Yellow Emperor's Internal Classic.*

Huangtingjing. *Yellow Courtyard Classics.*

huantiao. An acupuncture cavity located on the buttocks.

Hubei. A province in north China.

Hui-zong. A Chinese emperor during the Song dynasty.

huiyin. An acupuncture cavity located on the perineum.

huo. Fire.

Jixiao Xinshu. *The New Book of Effective Disciplines.*

Jian-wen. A Chinese emperor during the Ming dynasty.

Jiang Fa. A military officer during the latter part of the Ming dynasty.

Jian Hua Taijiquan. Simplified Taijiquan.

jin. Martial art's power.

jin. Metal.

kong qi. Air energy.

kung fu (gongfu). Martial arts: time and energy.

laogong. An acupuncture cavity located on the palm.

Li, Bo-kui. One of Chen, Chang-xing's students.

Li, Yi-yu. Student of Wǔ, Yu-xiang; author of *Taijiquan Brief* (AD 1832–1892).

Liang dynasty. A Chinese dynasty (AD 502–557).

Liang, Zhi-Xiang. Liang, Shou-Yu's grandfather.

Liang, Shou-Yu. Coauthor of *Simplified Tai Chi Chuan*.

Liuqinxi. *Six Animal Play.*

Lui An. Creator and author of *Six Animal Play*.

ma bu. Horse stance.

Ming dynasty. A Chinese dynasty (AD 1368–1644).

Ming Langying Qixiu Leigao. A Ming dynasty history book.

Ming, Tai-zu. A Chinese emperor during the Ming dynasty.

mingmen. An acupuncture cavity located on the back, near the fourteenth vertebra.

Mingshi Fangjizhuan. A Ming dynasty history book.

mu. Wood.

pu bu. Half squat stance.

qi (chi). Intrinsic substance of all things; energy.

Qi, Ji-guang, Marshal. Author of *Ji Xiao Xin Shu*.

qigong. Energy study, drill, training.

Qing (Ching) dynasty. A Chinese dynasty (AD 1644–1912).

Qingcheng Mountain. A mountain in Sichuan Province, China.

qin na (chin na). Seize and control techniques.

quan. Fist.

Quanjing Sanshier Shi. *Martial Classic in Thirty-Two Postures.*

ren qi. Human energy.

Ren-zong. A Chinese emperor during the Song dynasty.

san shi qi shi. Thirty-seven postures.

Shang dynasty. A Chinese dynasty (1766–1123 BC).

shang xia xiang sui. Upper and lower body follow each other.

Shangdong. A city in China.

Shanghai. A province in China.

Shanxi. A province in China.

Shaolin. A Chinese martial art system.

she qing ding shan ge. Tongue gently touches the roof of the mouth.

shen ti zhong zheng. Body centered and upright.

Shuai Jiao. A Chinese martial arts style: Chinese wrestling.

shui. Water.

Sichuan. A province in China.

Song dynasty. A Chinese dynasty (AD 960–1126).

song yao song kua. Loosen your waist and hips.

Sun, Lu-tang. Founder of the Sun Style Taijiquan.

Sun Style. One of the five major taijiquan styles.

taiji (tai chi). Grand ultimate.

taijiquan (tai chi chuan). The grand ultimate fist.

Taijiquan Xiaoxu. *Taijiquan Brief.*

Taiwan. Known as the Republic of China, it is an island separate from mainland China.

Tang dynasty. A Chinese dynasty (AD 618–906).

tian di yi da ren shen. Universe is a big human body.

tian qi. Heaven's energy; weather.

tian ren he yi. Heaven and humans combine as one.

tu. Earth.

tu gu na xin. Expel "old" air; inhale "new" air.

tu na. The art of breathing.

Wang, Ju-rong. Chinese martial arts expert; daughter of Wang, Zi-ping.

Wang, Wei-yi. The person responsible for charting the acupuncture Bronze Man.

Wang Zong. The Ming dynasty person once mistaken as Wang, Zon-yue of the Qing dynasty.

Wang, Zong-yue. Author of *Taijiquan Classic*.

Wanzhengnan Muzhiming. The book written by Huang, Li-zhou.

weilu zhong zheng. Sacrum centered and upright.

wu. Five.

Wu, Gong-zao. Second son of Wu, Jian-quan.

Wu, Gong-yi. First son of Wu, Jian-quan.

Wu, Jian-quan. Founder of Wu Style Taijiquan (AD 1870–1942).

Wu, Quan-you. Also known as Quan You, a Manchurian who learned Taijiquan from Yang, Lu-chan; father of Wu, Jaian-quan (AD 1834–1902).

Wu Style. One of the five major taijiquan styles.

Wŭ Style. One of the five major taijiquan styles.

Wu, Wen-Ching. Coauthor of *Simplified Tai Chi Chuan*.

Wu, Ying-hua. Daughter of Wu, Jian-quan.

Wŭ, Yu-xiang. Founder of Wŭ Style Taijiquan.

Wudang (Wutang) Mountain. A mountain in Hubei Province, China.

wuji. The beginning of the Dao (Tao), or the cosmos; the undifferentiated beginning.

Wuqinxi. *Five Animal Play,* by Dr. Hua Tuo.

wushu. Chinese martial arts.

wuxing. Five elements.

xiang cheng. Mutual overrestraint.

xiang ke. Mutual restraint.

xiang sheng. Mutual nourishment.

xiang wu. Mutual reverse restraint.

xiao jiu tian. Little nine heaven.

xie gong bu. Slant bow stance.

xie bu. Resting stance.

xin. Mind; heart.

xing. Behavior, conduct, or travel.

Xingyiquan. An internal Chinese martial art style.

xu ling ding jin. Vitality of spirit leads to the top of the head.

Xu Xi. The doctor who cured Emperor Ren-zong with acupuncture.

xu bu. Empty stance.

yang. Counterpart of yin.

Yang, Ban-hou. Second son of Yang, Lu-chan (AD 1837–1892).

Yang, Cheng-fu. Yang, Jian-hou's third son, and Yang, Lu-chan's grandson (AD 1883–1936).

Yang, Jian-hou. Yang, Lu-chan's third son (AD 1839–1917).

Yang, Jwing-Ming. Wu, Wen-Ching's teacher.

Yang, Lu-chan. Founder of Yang Style Taijiquan (AD 1799–1872).

Yang, Shao-hou. Yang, Jian-hou's oldest son, and Yang, Lu-chan's grandson (AD 1862–1930).

Yang Style. One of the five major taijiquan styles.

Yang, Zhen-duo. Yang, Cheng-fu's son, and Yang, Lu-chan's great grandson.

yang shen fa. Life-nourishing technique.

yan shen zhu shi. Eyes focus with concentration.

yi. Mind, intent.

yi shen yi xiao tian di. Chinese belief that translates as "human body is a small heaven and earth."

yi shou dan tian. Mind focuses at dan tian, your body's center of gravity.

yi yi ling qi. Use your mind to lead the qi.

Yi Chuan. Theoretical and philosophical explanations of *Yi Jing;* vol. 2 of *Zhouyi.*

Yi Jing (*I Ching*). *Book of Changes.*

yin. Counterpart of yang.

yin ti lingrou. Stretch the body to attain flexibility.

yin and yang. Philosophy used to explain the cosmos.

yin and yang dui li. Yin and yang opposition.

yin and yang hugen. Yin and yang interdependence.

yin and yang xiao zhang. Yin and yang decreasing and increasing.

yin and yang zhuan hua. Yin and yang transformation.

Yong-le. A Chinese emperor during the Ming dynasty.

yongquan. An acupuncture cavity on the bottom of the foot.

yuan jing. Original essence.

zhang. Palm.

Zhang, San-feng (Chang, San-feng). The legendary founder of taijiquan.

Zhaobao Style. A Taijiquan style.

zheng gong bu. Straight bow stance.

Zhongguo Tiyu Yundong Weiyuanhui. Chinese National Athletic Association.

Zhouyi. Zhou dynasty's *Book of Changes,* vol. 1, and *Yi Chuan,* vol. 2.

zi mu xiang ji. Mother-son mutual burdening.

zuo wan shen zhi. Extend the fingers and settle the wrist.

zuo bu. Sit back stance.

BIBLIOGRAPHY

Barrett, James M., Peter Abramoff, A. Krishna Kumaran, and William F. Millington. *Biology.* Englewood Cliffs, NJ: Prentice-Hall, 1986.

Chen, Yan-Lin. *Tai Ji Quan Dao Jian Gan San Shou He Bian* [Taijiquan, saber, sword, staff, and sparring]. Reprinted in Taipei, Taiwan: Jinchuan Publication Company, 1981.

Gu, Liu-Xin. *Chen Shi Tai Ji Pao Chui Quan* [Chen style tai chi cannon fist]. Reprinted in Taipei, Taiwan: Hualian Publication Company, 1985.

Kang, Ge-Wu. *Zhong Guo Wu Shu Shi Yong Da Quan* [Comprehensive collection of Chinese martial arts]. Reprinted in Taipei, Taiwan: Wuzhou Publication Company, 1979.

Lai, Ming and Tai-Yin Lin. *The New Lin Yutang Chinese-English Dictionary.* Hong Kong: Panorama Press Ltd., 1987.

Meng, Jing-Chun and Zhong-Ying Zhou. *Zhong Yi Xue Gai Lun* [An introduction to learn traditional Chinese medicine]. Taipei, Taiwan: Zhiyin Publication Company, 1991.

Yang, Cheng-Fu. *Yang Shi Tai Ji Fa: Yuan Zhu Yang Cheng-Fu.* [Yang Style Tai Chi Chuan, the correct way: The original work of Yang, Cheng-Fu]. Originally published 1934, no publication information available. Reprinted in Hong Kong: Wenhai Publication Company, 1986(?).

Yang, Jwing-Ming. *Advanced Yang Style Tai Chi Chuan.* vol. 1. Boston: YMAA Publication Center, Inc., 1987.

———. *The Root of Chinese Chi Kung.* Boston: YMAA Publication Center, Inc., 1989.

Yang, Li. *Zhou Yi Yu Zhong Yi Xue* [Book of changes and traditional Chinese medicine]. Taipei, Taiwan: Lequn Culture Enterprise Company, 1990.

Yang, Wei-Jie. *Huang Di Nei Jing Su Wen Shi Jie* [An explanation of the basic questions: Text of the Yellow Emperor's inner canon]. Taipei, Taiwan: Tailian Goufeng Publication Company, 1984.

ABOUT THE AUTHOR:
Master Liang, Shou-Yu

Master Liang, Shou-Yu was born in 1943 in Sichuan, China. At age six he began his training in *qigong* (the art of breathing and internal energy control), under the tutelage of his renowned grandfather, the late Liang, Zhi-Xiang. He was taught the esoteric skills of the Emei Mountain sect, including Dapeng Qigong. When he was eight, his grandfather made special arrangements for him to begin training Emei Wushu (martial arts).

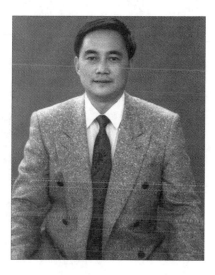

In 1959, as a young boy, Mr. Liang began the study of Qin Na (Chin Na) and Chinese Shuai Jiao (wrestling). From 1960 to 1964, he devoted his attention to the research and practice of wrestling and wushu.

Added to the advantage of being born to a traditional wushu family, Mr. Liang also had the opportunity of coming into contact with many legendary grandmasters. By the time he was twenty, Mr. Liang had already received instruction from ten of the best-known contemporary masters of both Southern and Northern origin. His curiosity inspired him to learn more than one hundred sequences from many different styles. His study of the martial arts has taken him throughout mainland China, including Henan Province to learn Chen Style Taijiquan (Tai Chi Chuan), Hubei Province to learn the Wudang (Wuudang) system, and Hunan Province to learn the Nanyue system.

With his wealth of knowledge, Mr. Liang was inspired to compete in martial arts competitions, in which he was many times a noted gold medalist. During his adolescence, Mr. Liang won titles in Chinese wrestling (Shuai Jiao), various other martial arts, and weight lifting.

As he grew older, through and beyond his college years, his wide background in various martial arts helped form his present character and led him to achieve a high level of martial skill. Some of the styles he concentrated on included the esoteric Emei system, Shaolin Long Fist, Praying Mantis, Chuo Jiao, Qin Na, vital point striking, many weapons systems, and several kinds of internal qigong.

Mr. Liang received a university degree in biology and physiology in 1964. However, during this time of political turmoil, and because of his bourgeois family background, the Communist government sent him to a remote, poverty-stricken village to teach high school. Despite this setback, Mr. Liang began to organize teams in wushu and wrestling.

Then came a disastrous time in modern Chinese history. During the years of the Cultural Revolution (1966–1974), all forms of martial arts and qigong were suppressed. Because he came from a bourgeois family, Mr. Liang was vulnerable to the furious passions and blind madness of the revolutionaries. To avoid conflict with the Red Guards, he gave up his teaching position and used this opportunity to tour the various parts of the country. During his travels, he visited and discovered great masters in wushu, and made friends with people who shared his devotion and love for the art. Mr. Liang went through numerous provinces and cities, visiting the many renowned and revered places where wushu originated, developed, and was refined. Among the many places he visited were Emei Mountain, Wudang Mountain, Hua Mountain, Qingcheng Mountain, Chen Village in Henan, the Changzhou Territory in Hebei Province, Beijing, and Shanghai. In eight years he made many wushu friends and met many great masters, and his mastery of the techniques and philosophy of the art grew to new horizons.

At the end of the Cultural Revolution, the Chinese government again began to support the martial arts and qigong, including competition. There was a general consensus that they should organize and categorize the existing external and internal martial arts. Research projects were set up to seek out the living old masters, select their best techniques, and organize their knowledge. It was at this time that the Sichuan government appointed Mr. Liang as a coach for the city, the territory, and the province. So many of his students were among the top martial artists of China that, in 1979, he was voted one of the top professional wushu coaches since 1949 by the People's Republic of China. Also, he often served as a judge in national competitions.

After the Cultural Revolution, despite his many official duties, Mr. Liang continued to participate actively in competitions both at the provincial and national levels. Between 1974 and 1981, he won numerous medals, including four gold medals. His students also performed superbly both in national and provincial open tournaments, winning many medals. Many of these students have now become professional wushu coaches, college wushu instructors, armed forces wushu trainers, and movie stars. In 1979, Mr. Liang received several appointments, including committee member of the Sichuan Chapter of the Chinese National Wushu Association and Coaches Committee.

When Mr. Liang first visited Seattle, Washington, in 1981, it marked a new era in the course of his life. His ability immediately impressed wushu devotees, and the

Wushu and Taiji Club of the Student Association at the University of Washington retained him as a wushu coach. At the same time, Mr. Liang was giving lessons at the Taiji Association in Seattle. In the following year, Mr. Liang went north to Vancouver, Canada, and was appointed taiji coach by the Villa Cathy Care Home. The same year, he was appointed honorary chairman and head coach by the North American Taiji Athletic Association.

In 1984, Mr. Liang was certified as a national first-class ranking judge by China. He was also appointed chairperson and wushu coach by the University of British Columbia. In 1985, Mr. Liang was elected coach of the First Canadian National Wushu Team, which was invited to participate in the First International Wushu Invitational Tournament that took place in Xian, China. The Canadian team won third place after competing against teams from thirteen other countries.

The following year, Mr. Liang was elected coach of the Second Canadian National Wushu Team, which competed in the Second International Wushu Invitational Tournament, held in Teintsin, China. A total of twenty-eight countries participated. This time, the Canadian team earned more medals than any other country, except the host country. Mr. Liang's role and achievements were reported in fourteen newspapers and magazines throughout China. The performances and demonstrations of the Canadian team and Mr. Liang were broadcast on the Sichuan television station.

Mr. Liang has not limited his contributions of taiji, wushu, and qigong to Canada. He has also given numerous seminars and demonstrations to students and instructors in the United States and Europe, including instructors and professionals from such disciplines as karate, taiji, and Shaolin Kung Fu. Students in Boston, Houston, Denver, New York, Pennsylvania, Georgia, Virginia, and Italy have benefited greatly from Mr. Liang's personal touch. Since the beginning of his glorious martial arts life, he has been featured by more than thirty newspapers and magazines in China, Europe, the US, and Canada, as well as being interviewed by several television stations in China, the US, and Canada. Mr. Liang has published instructional video programs teaching *Lian Gong Shi Ba Fa*, *24 Form Taijiquan*, and *Vital Hsing Yi Quan* and has coauthored a book, *Hsing Yi Chuan*.

ABOUT THE AUTHOR:
Mr. Wu, Wen-Ching

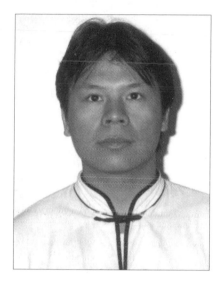

Mr. Wu was born in Taiwan, Republic of China, in 1964. In 1976, he went to West Africa with his family, where he attended an international school. Mr. Wu graduated as the salutatorian of his high school class.

In 1983, Mr. Wu went to Boston, Massachusetts, to attend Northeastern University. It was at this time that Mr. Wu was accepted by Dr. Yang as a student. Mr. Wu's dedicated training helped him excel in Shaolin Long Fist and White Crane Kung Fu as well as in Yang Style Taijiquan (Tai Chi Chuan). In five years, Mr. Wu completed the cooperative and academic requirements at Northeastern University and received his BSME degree, with honors, and also qualified as an assistant instructor under Dr. Yang.

After graduation, Mr. Wu began working as a mechanical engineer during the day and teaching Shaolin Kung Fu and taijiquan classes at YMAA Headquarters in the evenings. He also continued his advanced training under Dr. Yang's personal guidance.

After years of dedicated training, Mr. Wu proved his moral character and martial arts potential in both internal and external styles to Dr. Yang. In May 1989, Mr. Wu was publicly accepted by Dr. Yang as a disciple.

In 1986, Mr. Wu had the good fortune to be introduced to Master Liang, Shou-Yu by Dr. Yang. Mr. Wu's martial potential and moral character won the liking of Master Liang. For the last seven years Master Liang has willingly shared much of his vast knowledge with Mr. Wu. Mr. Wu has learned Xingyiquan, Baguazhang, White Ape Sword, and taijiquan from Master Liang.

With Dr. Yang and Master Liang's encouragement, Mr. Wu competed in eight events in the 1990 United States National Chinese Martial Arts Competition held in Houston, Texas. Mr. Wu was ranked first nationally in every event he competed in. He was awarded two of the highest medals in the competition: Men's All-Around Internal Style and External Style Grand Champion.

On November 6, 1990, with Dr. Yang's permission, Mr. Wu founded Yang's Martial Arts Association of Rhode Island (YMAA-RI) and continues to pass down his lineage of Chinese martial arts. In less than two years YMAA-RI established a solid foundation, attracting students from Rhode Island and neighboring states. During the past two years, Mr. Wu not only offered his expertise to students at YMAA-RI, but he has also traveled to several other states and countries to offer seminars on taijiquan, Xingyiquan, Baguazhang, and Shaolin Kung Fu. He was also featured on a cable talk show introducing taijiquan and its benefits to the audience. During this time, he also translated the major part of *Traditional Yang Family Style Taijiquan*, a video by the fourth- and sixth-generation Yang family descendants. It is his goal to carry on his teachers' legacies, not only by improving his own ability and understanding, but by benefiting others through his teaching and writing.

INDEX

BOOKS FROM YMAA

more products available from . . .
YMAA Publication Center, Inc. 楊氏東方文化出版中心

1-800-669-8892 • info@ymaa.com • www.ymaa.com

DVDS FROM YMAA

ADVANCED PRACTICAL CHIN NA IN-DEPTH

ANALYSIS OF SHAOLIN CHIN NA

BAGUAZHANG: EMEI BAGUAZHANG

CHEN STYLE TAIJIQUAN

CHIN NA IN-DEPTH COURSES 1–4

CHIN NA IN-DEPTH COURSES 5–8

CHIN NA IN-DEPTH COURSES 9–12

FACING VIOLENCE: 7 THINGS A MARTIAL ARTIST MUST KNOW

FIVE ANIMAL SPORTS

JOINT LOCKS

KNIFE DEFENSE: TRADITIONAL TECHNIQUES AGAINST A DAGGER

KUNG FU BODY CONDITIONING 1

KUNG FU BODY CONDITIONING 2

KUNG FU FOR KIDS

KUNG FU FOR TEENS

LOGIC OF VIOLENCE

NORTHERN SHAOLIN SWORD : SAN CAI JIAN, KUN WU JIAN, QI MEN JIAN

QIGONG MASSAGE

QIGONG FOR HEALING

QIGONG FOR LONGEVITY

QIGONG FOR WOMEN

SABER FUNDAMENTAL TRAINING

SANCHIN KATA: TRADITIONAL TRAINING FOR KARATE POWER

SHAOLIN KUNG FU FUNDAMENTAL TRAINING: COURSES 1 & 2

SHAOLIN LONG FIST KUNG FU: BASIC SEQUENCES

SHAOLIN LONG FIST KUNG FU: INTERMEDIATE SEQUENCES

SHAOLIN LONG FIST KUNG FU: ADVANCED SEQUENCES 1

SHAOLIN LONG FIST KUNG FU: ADVANCED SEQUENCES 2

SHAOLIN SABER: BASIC SEQUENCES

SHAOLIN STAFF: BASIC SEQUENCES

SHAOLIN WHITE CRANE GONG FU BASIC TRAINING: COURSES 1 & 2

SHAOLIN WHITE CRANE GONG FU BASIC TRAINING: COURSES 3 & 4

SHUAI JIAO: KUNG FU WRESTLING

SIMPLE QIGONG EXERCISES FOR ARTHRITIS RELIEF

SIMPLE QIGONG EXERCISES FOR BACK PAIN RELIEF

SIMPLIFIED TAI CHI CHUAN: 24 & 48 POSTURES

SUNRISE TAI CHI

SUNSET TAI CHI

SWORD: FUNDAMENTAL TRAINING

TAEKWONDO KORYO POOMSAE

TAI CHI BALL QIGONG: COURSES 1 & 2

TAI CHI BALL QIGONG: COURSES 3 & 4

TAI CHI CHUAN CLASSICAL YANG STYLE

TAI CHI CONNECTIONS

TAI CHI ENERGY PATTERNS

TAI CHI FIGHTING SET

TAI CHI PUSHING HANDS: COURSES 1 & 2

TAI CHI PUSHING HANDS: COURSES 3 & 4

TAI CHI SWORD: CLASSICAL YANG STYLE

TAI CHI SYMBOL: YIN YANG STICKING HANDS

TAIJI & SHAOLIN STAFF: FUNDAMENTAL TRAINING

TAIJI CHIN NA IN-DEPTH

TAIJI 37 POSTURES MARTIAL APPLICATIONS

TAIJI SABER CLASSICAL YANG STYLE

TAIJI WRESTLING

UNDERSTANDING QIGONG 1: WHAT IS QI? • HUMAN QI CIRCULATORY SYSTEM

UNDERSTANDING QIGONG 2: KEY POINTS • QIGONG BREATHING

UNDERSTANDING QIGONG 3: EMBRYONIC BREATHING

UNDERSTANDING QIGONG 4: FOUR SEASONS QIGONG

UNDERSTANDING QIGONG 5: SMALL CIRCULATION

UNDERSTANDING QIGONG 6: MARTIAL QIGONG BREATHING

WHITE CRANE HARD & SOFT QIGONG

WUDANG KUNG FU: FUNDAMENTAL TRAINING

WUDANG SWORD

WUDANG TAIJIQUAN

XINGYIQUAN

YANG TAI CHI FOR BEGINNERS

YMAA 25-YEAR ANNIVERSARY DVD

more products available from . . .

YMAA Publication Center, Inc. 楊氏東方文化出版中心

1-800-669-8892 • info@ymaa.com • www.ymaa.com